The Addictive Brain

Thad A. Polk, Ph.D.

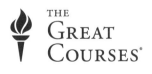

THE
GREAT
COURSES®

PUBLISHED BY:

THE GREAT COURSES
Corporate Headquarters
4840 Westfields Boulevard, Suite 500
Chantilly, Virginia 20151-2299
Phone: 1-800-832-2412
Fax: 703-378-3819
www.thegreatcourses.com

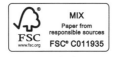

Thad A. Polk, Ph.D.

Arthur F. Thurnau Professor of Psychology
University of Michigan

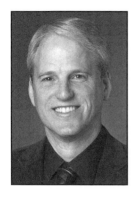

Professor Thad A. Polk is an Arthur F. Thurnau Professor in the Departments of Psychology and Electrical Engineering and Computer Science at the University of Michigan. He received a B.A. in Mathematics from the University of Virginia and an interdisciplinary Ph.D. in Computer Science and Psychology from Carnegie Mellon University. He received postdoctoral training in cognitive neuroscience at the University of Pennsylvania before joining the faculty at the University of Michigan.

Professor Polk's research combines functional imaging of the human brain with computational modeling and behavioral methods to investigate the neural architecture underlying cognition. Some of his major projects have investigated differences in the brains of smokers who quit compared with those who do not, changes in the brain as we age, and contributions of nature versus nurture to neural organization. Professor Polk regularly collaborates with scientists at the University of Texas at Dallas and at the Max Planck Institute for Human Development in Berlin, where he is a frequent visiting scientist. At the University of Michigan, he is a cochair of the Department of Psychology and the chair of the Health Sciences and Behavioral Sciences Institutional Review Boards.

Professor Polk regularly teaches large lecture courses as well as small seminars on topics ranging from the human mind and brain, to cognitive psychology, to computational modeling of cognition. His teaching at the University of Michigan has been recognized by numerous awards, including the Excellence in Education Award from the College of Literature, Science, and the Arts and the Arthur F. Thurnau Professorship, the university's highest undergraduate teaching award. He also was featured in the University of Michigan's Professors Reaching Out for Students (PROFS) lecture series and was named to The Princeton Review's list of the Best 300 Professors in the United States. ∎

Table of Contents

Table of Contents

Acknowledgments

I'd like to thank the following individuals, whose scholarship, advice, and assistance greatly contributed to the preparation of the lectures for this Great Course.

First, I'd like to thank Dr. Joshua Berke, whose outstanding lectures on drugs of abuse at the University of Michigan provided many ideas for how best to explain how different drugs work. I'd also like to thank Dr. Jerrold Meyer and Dr. Linda Quenzer, whose outstanding book *Psychopharmacology: Drugs, the Brain, and Behavior* served as a central reference for the lectures on individual drugs.

My colleagues Dr. Kent Berridge, Dr. Terry Robinson, and Dr. Ashley Gearhardt at the University of Michigan, who are experts in the field of addiction, generously provided very helpful input on the lectures covering the neuroscience of addiction and junk food addiction.

I'd also like to express my gratitude to the many students at Michigan who provided feedback and fact-checking on earlier versions of the lectures for this course, including Serene Mirza, Chloe Yang, Dana Abufarha, Ian Bernstein, Brianna Campbell, Sam Cass, Jordan Chamberlain, Jordan Chick, Gina Goldfaden, Dustin Hartz, Steven Levenbrook, Kiara Marshall, Nadir Rehman, John Rose, Allison Vogel, Tommy Wydra, Tanmayee Yenumula, and Brandon Yousif.

Finally, I'd like to thank my wife, Norma, and my three daughters—Sarah, Rachel, and Lydia—for putting up with me while I was devoting every spare minute to working on this course!

The Addictive Brain

Scope:

Addiction is a modern-day epidemic. More than 500 people die every hour as a result of an addiction-related disease or an overdose, and addiction is estimated to cost the United States more than 600 billion dollars every year in health-care costs, lost productivity, and crime. Families are destroyed, careers are lost, and lives are wasted. And the problem is only getting worse. If we ever hope to stem the tide, it is imperative that we develop a better understanding of what addiction is and how it works at a neural level. Fortunately, scientists have made significant progress in answering these questions in the last few decades. This course will survey this important and exciting field.

The course begins by providing some fundamental background on addiction, its relatively recent rise in prevalence, and the scope of the problem today. It then turns to one of the most important discoveries in the science of addiction—namely, that all addictions hijack the brain's natural reward system, leading to an almost-irresistible urge to pursue the object of the addiction. The normal operation of the reward system, the way it is changed in addiction, and the crucial role of dopamine—the so-called addiction molecule—will all be covered in depth. The course will also explain the genetics of addiction and explore why some people are significantly more susceptible to addiction than others.

The second major section of the course will focus on drugs. One lecture will explain how certain drugs can produce psychological effects by mimicking the brain's own chemical messengers, the neurotransmitters. Then, a sequence of lectures will cover caffeine, nicotine, alcohol, marijuana, opioids like heroin, and stimulants like cocaine and methamphetamine. These lectures will explain in detail how these drugs work and how their chronic use can lead to dependence and addiction.

The final section of the course will discuss so-called behavioral addictions, such as pathological gambling, food addiction, and video game addiction. These lectures will explore evidence that these stimuli are supernormal in the sense that they activate the brain's reward system significantly more than other stimuli do, resulting in addictions similar to those seen with drugs of abuse.

By the end of this course, you will have a new understanding of what's going on in the brains of alcoholics, crack addicts, smokers, and adolescents hooked on video games. And that understanding will make you a more informed consumer of the many stories about addiction in the popular press. You also will be in a much better position to form an educated opinion about controversial topics surrounding addiction, such as whether addiction is a disease and how our society should respond to the growing problem of addiction today. ■

Addiction 101

Lecture 1

Addiction affects almost all of us. This course will present scientific findings about addiction in a relatively objective way. This lecture will provide some background on drugs and addiction. You also will learn about the history of drug use and the war on drugs, as well as the societal and personal impacts of drug addiction. The goal of this course is to help you develop a better understanding of addiction, how it works, and how it manages to take hold of so many people around the world.

Drugs

- A drug is typically considered to be a substance other than food that changes biological functioning when it's introduced into the body from outside. Cocaine, heroin, and marijuana all satisfy this definition, but so do antacids and antibiotics—so what's the difference?

- One of the key differences is that cocaine and heroin are psychoactive while antacids and antibiotics are not. Psychoactive drugs affect the function of the brain and produce psychological effects like changes in mood, perception, and cognition. Psychoactive drugs are often addictive. Psychoactive drugs are not limited to the hard drugs like cocaine and heroin. Nicotine, alcohol, and caffeine are also psychoactive drugs.

- Using a psychoactive drug is different than being addicted to a psychoactive drug. In fact, many potentially addictive psychoactive drugs are used in modern medicine every day without any problems. For example, stimulant drugs like Ritalin and Adderall are very commonly used in the treatment of attention deficit/hyperactivity disorder despite the fact that they're potentially addictive when used inappropriately.

- Likewise, opioid drugs like morphine and codeine can be very addictive, but they're still the drugs of choice in the management of pain. And when implemented as directed by a physician, these treatments don't usually lead to addiction.

- Furthermore, millions of people use psychoactive drugs recreationally from time to time, and the vast majority of them aren't addicted, either—nor do they become addicted. Consider the huge number of people who drink alcohol on a regular basis without becoming alcoholics, for example.

Addiction

- What constitutes a real addiction? It turns out that answering this question is tricky. In fact, many scientists try to avoid using the term "addiction" entirely, because the word can mean different things to different people. As a result, psychiatrists often prefer the term "substance use disorder" to make clear that the behavior in question is actually abnormal and unhealthy.

- Substance use disorders are diagnosed based on the presence of a subset of 11 characteristic features. If two or three of the characteristic features are present, then a mild addiction is diagnosed. If four or five features are present, then a moderate addiction is diagnosed. And the presence of six or more features indicates a severe addiction.

- The characteristic features can be divided into three groups: those related to abuse, dependence, and craving. First, consider abuse. For behavior to be considered an addiction, it has to lead to significant negative consequences for the addict. Some of those consequences might be physical. For example, alcoholics often continue drinking despite significant liver damage. Or the negative consequences might be social and interpersonal. Many addicts continue in their addictive behavior to the point that it alienates friends and family. Furthermore, addicts often end up neglecting major responsibilities as a result of their habit.

- Another hallmark feature of addiction is dependence. Drug addicts often get to the point that they depend on their drug, both psychologically and even physically. One of the main symptoms of physical dependence is the development of tolerance to the effects of a drug. Addicts often need more of the drug to get the effect that they want. Another symptom of physical dependence is withdrawal. If a drug addict abruptly quits taking their drug, they'll often experience very unpleasant physical and psychological symptoms. In fact, many addicts will tell you that they actually need to take their drugs just to feel normal; they just don't function properly without them.

- The third hallmark feature of addiction is craving. When they're not using, drug addicts often report an extremely strong desire or urge to use their drug. This craving can be so strong that the addict may find it difficult to think about anything else; he or she becomes completely obsessed with getting more of the drug. Furthermore, environmental cues that are associated with drug use become very strong triggers for craving. For example, a heroin addict's cravings might be triggered by seeing a needle.

- Scientists have discovered some fascinating evidence that suggests that it is possible to be addicted to something other than a drug. For example, pathological gambling satisfies many of the major criteria of addiction. It, too, is characterized by craving and by persistent, compulsive behavior despite significant negative consequences. So, many scientists now consider so-called behavioral or process addictions like gambling to be the same kind of addictive disorder as chronic drug abuse.

The History of Drug Use and the War on Drugs
- Roughly 80 million Americans could be considered addicts. But while addiction has only recently become a major threat, drugs are not new, and drug use is not a modern development. Most of the drugs that people commonly use and abuse today are derived from plants, and people have recognized the psychological and physiological effects of those plants for thousands of years.

- There is evidence that by the year 3400 B.C., the Sumerians were aware of the psychological effects of the opium poppy, from which opium and heroin are derived. Likewise, South Americans have chewed coca leaves, containing cocaine, for millennia. And evidence from pottery jars in China suggests that people have been drinking alcohol since at least 7000 B.C.

- Nevertheless, drug addiction has become much more of a problem in the last 150 years than it ever was before. And one possible reason is that about 200 years ago, people began isolating the active ingredients that produced the psychological and physiological effects associated with these plants. They were therefore able to make much more-potent forms of the drugs than had ever existed before.

- For example, in the early 1800s, scientists isolated morphine from opium, and a few decades later, they synthesized heroin from morphine. In 1859, cocaine was isolated from coca leaves. And alcohol had long been produced in more potent forms by the process of distillation.

- Some of these developments actually represented major medical breakthroughs. In particular, physicians finally had relatively pure drugs that were much more effective than anything they had before. For example, morphine provided very effective pain relief for soldiers injured in the Civil War. In fact, morphine is still the gold-standard painkiller in medicine today.

- When these addictive drugs first became widely available in the 1800s, they were completely unregulated. They were sold as miracle cures by traveling salesmen and could be purchased from catalogs through the mail. Morphine-based syrups were often used to treat teething pain in infants, heroin was sold as a cough suppressant, and cocaine was used as a core ingredient in a popular elixir.

- In the early 20th century, the first skirmishes in the war on drugs began in the United States. In 1906, Theodore Roosevelt signed into law the Pure Food and Drug Act, the first federal law regulating drugs and food. Although drugs like cocaine and heroin could still be sold as ingredients in products, the law required truth in labeling. Products containing these kinds of drugs had to be labeled as such. And improperly labeled products could be seized and destroyed at the manufacturer's expense.

- In 1914, the Harrison Narcotics Tax Act required anyone selling or giving away products containing substantial doses of cocaine or opium to register with what we would call today the Internal Revenue Service. It also made opium itself available only by prescription.

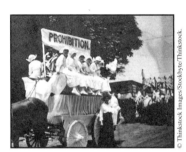

- And then came Prohibition. In 1917, the U.S. Senate proposed the 18th Amendment to the Constitution, which banned the sale and production of alcoholic drinks. The amendment was ratified in 1919 and went into effect on January 17, 1920. But Prohibition was extremely

With the controversial Prohibition movement came the 18th Amendment, which banned the production and sale of alcoholic beverages.

controversial, and a huge number of people continued drinking in spite of the law. And in 1933, the 18th Amendment became the only constitutional amendment ever to be repealed.

- In 1934, the Uniform State Narcotics Act brought the ever-growing number of state laws restricting narcotics into alignment. It also included measures to strengthen their enforcement, although that remained the responsibility of the states.

- The 1960s saw a revolution in social norms and the rise of a new antiestablishment counterculture in the United States. This was the era of the hippie movement, psychedelic rock, and the sexual revolution. And a very significant part of this counterculture was the free use of recreational drugs, particularly marijuana, LSD, and psychedelic mushrooms.

- In the early 1970s, President Richard Nixon signed into law the Controlled Substances Act, which was part of an attempt to create a unified and comprehensive federal drug policy. The act strictly classified which types of drugs were to be regulated, restricted, or banned outright, and it created two federal agencies—the Food and Drug Administration and the Drug Enforcement Administration—to implement these regulations. It was at this point that the United States openly declared an official war on drugs.

- And that war rages on, although with roughly 80 million addicts in the United States alone, it appears that we're losing. And the consequences are quite grave—economically, medically, and personally.

Societal and Personal Impacts of Drug Addiction

- Consider the economic impact that drug addiction has in the United States, for example.
  - The National Institute on Drug Abuse estimates that the abuse of tobacco, alcohol, and illicit drugs costs the United States about 600 billion dollars per year in costs related to crime, lost work productivity, and health care.

  - In terms of overall costs, alcohol abuse is the worst offender. It's estimated to cost about 235 billion dollars per year, which includes increased costs of health care due to the treatment of alcoholism, significant productivity losses in jobs, and property damage due to crimes and automobile crashes, among many other consequences.

- The abuse of tobacco and illicit drugs are each estimated to cost nearly 200 billion dollars per year. For tobacco, about half of that cost is due to the substantial price of health care for tobacco-related illnesses. For illicit drugs, a large proportion of the cost is related to crime and the criminal justice system.

- And, of course, those are just the economic costs. The costs in terms of human lives are much more tragic. For example, smoking-related illnesses are estimated to kill over 5 million people worldwide each year. Alcohol is involved in about half of all highway deaths, and the number of deaths due to drug overdose now exceeds the number of vehicle-related deaths in 29 states.

- Furthermore, about a quarter of intravenous drug users in the United States are infected with the AIDS virus, typically due to sharing dirty needles. Drug use is also associated with a significantly higher incidence of other sexually transmitted diseases, such as syphilis and gonorrhea.

- More personally, most of us know people whose lives have been touched by an addiction. Or maybe you are struggling with an addiction that you just haven't been able to kick. The truth is that addiction touches virtually all of us, directly or indirectly.

Suggested Reading

Conyers, *Addict in the Family*.

Escohotado, *A Brief History of Drugs*.

Johnson, ed., *Addiction Medicine*.

National Institute on Drug Abuse, *Drugs, Brains, and Behavior*.

Research Triangle Institute, "National Survey on Drug Use and Health."

Sheff, *Clean*.

1. What are the major characteristics of addiction?

2. What are some of the major milestones in the history of U.S. drug policy?

3. Why do you think addiction is so much more of a problem today than it was 200 years ago?

Lecture 1: Addiction 101

The Psychology and Neuroscience of Reward
Lecture 2

How do we learn from experiencing rewards or pleasures, and how does that experience reinforce the behaviors that led to that reward? This lecture will approach this question from two angles. First, you will learn about the psychology of reward processing, starting with Pavlov's famous dogs. Then, you will learn about the neuroscience of reward processing, along with some controversial experiments that attempted to locate the brain's pleasure centers. As you will discover, these two lines of research have recently converged in remarkable ways to provide new insights into the connections between how our minds and our brains process rewards.

The Psychology of Reward Processing

- Ivan Pavlov's study on classical conditioning in dogs is a famous experiment. Pavlov had developed an experimental setup in which he could collect saliva directly from the salivary glands of dogs when they smelled or saw food. But Pavlov noticed something unusual when he measured the output of saliva: The dogs were salivating as soon as he or his assistants entered the room, even though the dogs couldn't see or smell any food yet. Pavlov became interested in this phenomenon and began studying it directly.

- For example, he tried ringing a bell before the food was presented. The first time he rang the bell, the dogs didn't salivate. But if he consistently rang the bell before the food was presented, then pretty soon the dogs would associate that bell with food. Then, he could just ring the bell and the dog would salivate even if there wasn't any food present. This is the phenomenon of classical conditioning.

- One early explanation of Pavlov's conditioning results was based simply on co-occurrence: Maybe what's happening is that the bell and the food co-occur in time, and whenever stimuli co-occur like that, they become associated. Furthermore, the more frequently they're presented together, the stronger the association becomes. Sure enough, Pavlov found that if you present the bell with the food more frequently, then the association does become stronger.

- Subsequent experiments posed problems for this simple co-occurrence explanation, however. Suppose that you've conditioned a dog to strongly associate a bell with food. But now imagine that you start presenting another stimulus at the same time as the bell, such as making a salute—and only then do you present the dog with food. And you do this every time: Ring the bell, make a salute, and then give the dog food.

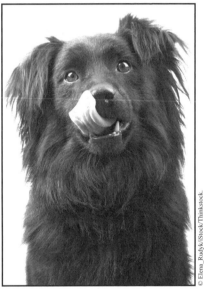

- Will the salute become associated with the food, too? Specifically, after enough training, will the act of saluting lead to salivation even without the sound of the bell? A simple co-occurrence explanation would predict that it would. But it turns out that this prediction is wrong.

- Once the dogs learned a strong association between the bell and the food, other stimuli that occurred with the bell did not become associated with the food. Saluting did

Pavlov found that he could condition dogs to salivate by consistently ringing a bell before presenting them with food.

not lead to salivation if the bell was missing. This phenomenon is referred to as blocking, and simple co-occurrence theories have a hard time explaining it.

- So, if a co-occurrence explanation is wrong, then what is going on? In 1972, psychologists Robert Rescorla and Allan Wagner proposed an answer that has become one of the most influential theories in all of psychology. Their so-called Rescorla-Wagner model was based on the idea that learning isn't based on co-occurrence but instead on prediction error.

- The idea of prediction error is that if you can already predict that the food is coming, then there's no real reason to change. You already know what you need to know, so there's not really an opportunity to learn something new. On the other hand, if the food shows up when you weren't predicting it—in other words, if you've made a prediction error—then that's a situation where you really want to learn so that you can make better predictions in the future.

- In the Rescorla-Wagner model, when an unexpected reward like food shows up, the stimuli that were present before its arrival begin to become more strongly associated with that reward. For example, the first few times the food shows up after the bell, the dogs probably weren't expecting it, so the association between the bell and the food is strengthened. But pretty soon, the dogs have developed a strong association between the bell and the food; they know what's coming. So, there's no need to change the association anymore because their prediction is accurate.

- Consider what the model would predict in the situation that led to blocking. The dogs had already been conditioned to expect the food after hearing the bell, but now an additional stimulus, such as a salute, gets paired with the bell. But the dogs are still predicting that the food will appear after the bell, and that prediction is accurate. So, there isn't any prediction error, and there's no need for additional learning. As a result, they don't learn an association between saluting and food. That association is blocked.

- Learning from prediction error plays a major role in modern artificial intelligence in a field called reinforcement learning, which involves figuring out how to behave in order to maximize long-term reward. In most situations, a sequence of multiple events precedes a reward. For example, the reward of winning chess or checkers requires a long sequence of actions that slowly move you closer to the goal.

- If you're learning chess and you stumble upon a sequence of moves that leads to an unexpected victory, the unexpected success constitutes a prediction error, so learning will occur, and the final action that led to that success will be reinforced. Furthermore, that prediction error can also be backed up and associated with the earlier actions that you took that led you to the final action. And now those actions can also be reinforced more than they already were.

- This is still prediction error learning, but it's prediction error learning over time, which is sometimes called temporal difference learning. Prediction error learning has now been used by countless artificial intelligence systems to learn a wide variety of complex behaviors.

The Neuroscience of Reward Processing
- In the 1950s, Robert Heath performed some controversial experiments on psychiatric patients. Heath implanted electrodes in their brains, and the electrodes were connected to a box with buttons that would stimulate particular regions of the patient's brain. The patients could actually stimulate their own brains by pressing a button.

- When the electrodes were implanted in a deep midline part of the brain called the septal region, the patients reported feeling pleasure and even excitement whenever the electrode was stimulated. In fact, they would repeatedly press the button more than 1,000 times and even complained when the box was taken away, asking for just a few more button presses. Stimulating the septal region also has been found to be chosen over sleep, taking care of children, and sex. This sounds a lot like addiction.

- Brain structures in and near the septal region are part of a neural circuit that plays a crucial role in processing reward and in motivating us to pursue reward. In addition to playing a central role in motivating normal behaviors like eating, the brain's reward circuit also plays a crucial role in the pathological behavior of addiction.

- There are three main components of the brain that are involved in processing reward: the nucleus accumbens, the prefrontal cortex, and the ventral tegmental area.

- The nucleus accumbens is often referred to as the brain's pleasure center. This is one of the regions that both humans and rats repeatedly stimulate to the exclusion of everything else in self-stimulation studies. It's located above and just behind your sinuses, near the midline of the brain. This region has been associated with a wide range of pleasures.

- The second major brain area involved in processing reward is the prefrontal cortex. The cerebral cortex, the gray matter on the outside of the brain, is often divided into four lobes: the occipital lobe at the back of the brain, the temporal lobe behind the ears, the parietal lobe at the top of the brain, and the frontal lobe at the front of the brain. The front part of the frontal lobe is called the prefrontal cortex, and it plays a central role in processing reward and controlling addictive behavior. It is often described as the CEO of the brain, because it sets goals and makes sure that they are accomplished.

- The third major brain region involved in processing reward is the ventral tegmental area (VTA), which is in the midbrain, at the top of the brain stem—the most primitive part of the brain. The VTA is located very near the middle of the head just slightly above the ears, a few inches behind and a little below the nucleus accumbens. Brain cells in the VTA project to both the nucleus accumbens and the prefrontal cortex and can therefore influence both pleasure and self-control. But what's most interesting about these cells is when they fire and when they don't.

- Wolfram Schultz and his colleagues performed some of the most influential studies of these cells at the University of Fribourg in Switzerland. They implanted electrodes in the VTA of monkeys so that they could record neural activity while the monkey was performing different tasks. Schultz proposed that activity in the VTA neurons reflects reward prediction error. When the neurons fire, it doesn't necessarily mean that a reward has arrived; rather, it means that there has been a reward prediction error.

- Prediction error is what the Rescorla-Wagner model used to signal a need for new learning. So, there is a convergence between the psychology of reward processing and the neuroscience of reward processing. But the convergence goes even further than that. In addition to learning based on prediction errors, temporal difference learning backs up that prediction error to previous stimuli or actions. And that's exactly what Schultz observed in VTA neurons.

- So, there is a very close correspondence between the temporal difference algorithm and the activity of neurons in the VTA. And artificial intelligence has demonstrated that temporal difference learning is extremely general, powerful, and effective, so it makes sense that the brain would be using a very similar approach.

- This convergence of the brain evidence with the psychological evidence has led many neuroscientists to conclude that prediction error learning, and specifically temporal difference learning, may be one of the fundamental mechanisms of learning in the brain. Furthermore, this type of reinforcement learning from prediction error is now widely believed to play a central role in the neuroscience of addiction.

Suggested Reading

Kringelbach and Berridge, "The Joyful Mind."

Nolte, *The Human Brain*.

Powell, Honey, and Symbaluk, *Introduction to Learning and Behavior*.

Schultz, Dayan, and Montague, "A Neural Substrate of Prediction and Reward."

Sutton and Barto, *Reinforcement Learning*.

Questions to Consider

1. How did the Rescorla-Wagner model differ from co-occurrence theories of classical conditioning?

2. What advance did temporal difference learning make relative to basic prediction error learning?

3. How would you describe the function of the nucleus accumbens, the prefrontal cortex, and the ventral tegmental area in motivated behavior?

How Addiction Hijacks the Brain
Lecture 3

In this lecture, you will learn about what is going on in the brain's reward system following chronic drug use and how that can lead to addiction. Along the way, you will link what you have learned so far about addiction with what you have learned so far about the brain. In addition, you will learn how behavioral symptoms such as tolerance, withdrawal, and dependence develop as a result of changes that occur in the brain.

Numbed Pleasure Response

- What does repeated use of addictive drugs like cocaine and alcohol do to the brain that makes them addictive? How does the brain change? There are three major changes that contribute to addiction: Repeated overstimulation of the brain's reward circuit numbs the response in the brain's pleasure center, the nucleus accumbens; repeated overstimulation also strengthens associations with addiction-related cues, which increases cravings; and it weakens inhibition from the prefrontal cortex, which undermines self-control.

- The first major change is the numbing of the pleasure response in the nucleus accumbens. Many scientists believe that tolerance reflects the brain's attempt to compensate for repeated overstimulation of the reward circuit and that it does so by inhibiting the stimulation of the nucleus accumbens, thereby numbing the pleasure response.

- The nucleus accumbens is often considered to be the pleasure center of the brain. It's associated with liking, or enjoyment. Direct stimulation of this area is so pleasurable that both rats and humans will self-stimulate it over and over for hours if given the opportunity.

- Addictive drugs stimulate the nucleus accumbens much more directly than normal, everyday rewards do, producing the extremely rewarding high associated with these drugs. Addictive drugs overstimulate the nucleus accumbens, meaning that they produce activity levels that are well beyond the normal range. If this kind of overstimulation happens a lot, it can eventually lead to a numbed pleasure response, because the nucleus accumbens will begin to inhibit the brain regions that are stimulating it.

- The body has mechanisms that maintain an internal equilibrium. This is called homeostasis. If the nucleus accumbens is repeatedly overstimulated, it will turn down the stimulation that it's receiving. It does this by producing a molecule called CREB, which triggers the production of dynorphin, which inhibits the stimulation of the nucleus accumbens.

- In a drug addict who is repeatedly overstimulating the nucleus accumbens with his or her drug of choice, the dynorphin will keep turning down the stimulation, and over time, the addict will feel less pleasure from the drug. The high won't be as rewarding. And the addict will require more and more stimulation to get the same level of reward. Eventually, the addict needs to take the drug just to feel normal. This is what is meant by a numbing of the pleasure response.

- The nucleus accumbens is becoming less sensitive to all types of stimulation, not just stimulation from addictive drugs. Everyday pleasures, such as seeing a friend or reading a book, might also feel numb. They won't provide the same level of pleasure they once did. In fact, because everyday pleasures don't activate the nucleus accumbens as directly or as strongly as drugs do, addicts can eventually reach a point where the drug is the only way they can feel good.

Strengthened Associations between Drug Taking and Drug-Related Cues

- The second major brain change that contributes to addiction is the strengthening of associations between drug taking and drug-related cues, resulting in increased craving. Addiction is characterized by very strong cravings and by compulsive use despite negative consequences.

- Where do these overwhelming cravings come from? First, it's important to note that craving or wanting is different from liking. This distinction is often particularly clear in drug addicts. Liking occurs in the nucleus accumbens, and the nucleus accumbens is getting numb. As this process occurs, how much drug addicts *like* the drugs declines over time. But how much they *want* the drugs doesn't. In fact, drug cravings tend to increase even though the pleasure derived from the drug is declining.

- If activity in the nucleus accumbens is associated with liking, what's the neural basis of wanting or craving? To answer that question, we need to turn to the ventral tegmental area (VTA) of the brain. Activity in the VTA is associated with reward prediction error; neurons in the VTA fire when a reward is unexpected.

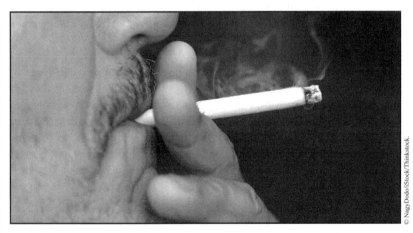

© Nagy Dodo/iStock/Thinkstock.

Addiction is characterized by very strong cravings and by compulsive use despite negative consequences.

- When VTA neurons fire, they release a chemical neurotransmitter called dopamine, which plays a central role in addiction. In fact, dopamine is so important that it's been called the addiction molecule. Studies have repeatedly found that all drugs of abuse lead to a significant increase in dopamine when they're taken. Dopamine seems to play a role in every addiction that's been studied, whether it's addiction to alcohol, cocaine, cigarettes, or even gambling.

- For a long time, scientists assumed that dopamine was associated with pleasure and liking, but recent evidence has suggested that that view is wrong. Evidence comes from patients with Parkinson's disease, which is associated with damage to cells in the midbrain that produce dopamine. Parkinson's patients have abnormally low levels of dopamine, and because dopamine also plays a major role in motor control, Parkinson's patients typically exhibit movement-related problems.

- But even though these patients have low levels of dopamine and associated motor problems, they still experience normal levels of pleasure. So, it appears that dopamine is not about pleasure or liking. Many scientists now believe that dopamine release is associated with wanting or craving, rather than liking. This kind of wanting or craving is an impulsive urge, not a thoughtful long-term goal.

- Kent Berridge and Terry Robinson at the University of Michigan refer to this kind of craving as incentive salience. That is, the incentive— or the motivation, or the wanting—becomes particularly salient and strong, and the dopamine signal conveys that strong incentive.

- The most compelling evidence that dopamine is associated with incentive salience, or this primitive kind of wanting, comes from studies with mice that have been genetically engineered to have abnormally high levels of dopamine. These dopamine-rich mice exhibit signs of very strong craving. For example, they move much more quickly toward rewarding stimuli like food than normal mice do. However, once they get the reward, they don't seem to enjoy it any more than the other mice, judging from their facial expressions.

- Even more interesting is the behavior of animals that have been genetically engineered not to produce dopamine. These animals don't show any motivation to try to obtain food or other rewards. In fact, they'll starve to death rather than taking the trouble to walk to the food. They actually have to be nursed in order to eat. But even though they don't show any signs of wanting the food, if the food is fed to them, they show all the normal facial expressions associated with liking the food.

- How does dopamine contribute to addiction? Repeated use of addictive drugs leads to changes in the dopamine system that contribute to addiction. There are at least two changes in the dopamine system that can contribute to addiction: The first change is what Robinson and Berridge call incentive sensitization, and the second change is related to dopamine's effect on associative learning.

- Robinson and Berridge proposed that with repeated use of addictive drugs, the brain's dopamine system becomes sensitized—that is, it becomes even more sensitive and easier to activate than it was before. Sensitization is kind of the opposite of tolerance. So, with repeated use of addictive drugs, the dopamine system responds more and more strongly.

- Dopamine is associated with craving or wanting. As the dopamine system becomes more and more sensitized, the cravings are becoming stronger and stronger. So, after the first few times of trying an addictive drug, the user might feel some urge to do it again, but those urges may not be particularly strong, and they can be resisted. But with repeated use, the dopamine system becomes sensitized, so the cravings become stronger and stronger, and pretty soon the urges are so strong that they're virtually irresistible.

- The other change involves dopamine's effect on associative learning. Recall that the Rescorla-Wagner model of classical conditioning is based on learning from prediction errors. Likewise, the temporal difference learning algorithm in artificial intelligence is based on reward prediction errors.

- Many scientists believe that dopamine is that reward prediction error. And, as such, it triggers learning just like prediction errors trigger learning in the Rescorla-Wagner model and the temporal difference algorithm. Essentially, when dopamine is released, it means that an unexpected reward has arrived, or soon will arrive. And that means that we should pay attention and learn so that we'll be able to predict when such rewards might show up again in the future.

- This makes a lot of sense and normally works really well. The release of dopamine signals that something important has happened, which leads to learning. Addictive drugs also trigger the release of dopamine, so they trigger learning, too. In fact, they trigger larger-than-normal releases of dopamine and therefore produce particularly strong learning. Unfortunately, what gets learned is more harmful than helpful.

- In any addict—whether the addiction is to alcohol, cocaine, nicotine, or any other addictive substance—certain environmental cues become very strongly associated with the use of the drug and turn into triggers that lead to craving and continued use.

Reduced Self-Control

- The third type of brain change that happens in addiction is reduced self-control as a result of weaker inhibitory control from the prefrontal cortex. The prefrontal cortex plays an important role in inhibiting undesirable behavior and in exerting self-control.

- While the reward circuit is mainly about processing primitive urges, the prefrontal cortex is the thinking part of the brain that can consider future consequences and make rational decisions about what actions we should take, not just what actions we feel like taking.

- And the prefrontal cortex plays a major role in inhibiting behavior suggested by the more primitive reward circuit, whenever we decide that that behavior wouldn't be appropriate. Unfortunately, chronic use of addictive drugs can lead to abnormalities in the prefrontal cortex that undermine our ability to exhibit this kind of self-control.

- For example, studies with rats have found that using cocaine for a month changes the structure of prefrontal neurons. In particular, the dendrites of the neurons (which receive inputs to the neuron) were misshapen in those animals compared with control animals. Likewise, neuroimaging studies in humans have found reduced activity in prefrontal cortex in chronic drug users compared with controls. In fact, even the volume of prefrontal cortex is reduced in drug addicts.

- Drug addicts also exhibit many of the same cognitive impairments that patients with damage to the prefrontal cortex exhibit. For example, prefrontal patients typically perform poorly on tasks of working memory and decision making, as well as on tasks that require sustained attention. And chronic drug users have been found to exhibit these same cognitive impairments.

- There is now quite a bit of evidence that chronic drug use impairs prefrontal cortex function. The problem is that the prefrontal cortex is the logical, rational circuit that understands consequences and that inhibits inappropriate behavior, but with repeated drug use, it doesn't work as well as it normally does and therefore has a hard time overcoming the increasingly powerful urges coming from the reward circuit. Essentially, the drug addict's ability to exhibit self-control and override drug craving becomes weaker and weaker.

Suggested Reading

Erickson, *The Science of Addiction*.

Everitt and Robbins. "Neural Systems of Reinforcement for Drug Addiction."

Nestler and Malenka, "The Addicted Brain."

Redish, *The Mind within the Brain*.

1. How would you characterize the positive and negative reinforcement models of addiction?

2. What are some of the major neural changes that occur with chronic drug use that contribute to addiction?

3. Based on what you've learned, do you think that addiction is a disease, a moral failure, or both?

Genetics—Born to Be an Addict?
Lecture 4

W   hy do some people get addicted while others don't? Can our genetic makeup make us more susceptible to addiction? And if so, how? These are the kinds of questions that will be addressed in this lecture. In this lecture, you will be introduced to what genes are, and you will learn about how geneticists have searched for genes that contribute to addiction susceptibility. You also will learn what geneticists have learned about what these susceptibility genes do, by analyzing studies using genetically engineered mice.

The Genetics of Addiction

- Studies have shown that certain people are innately more susceptible to addiction than others. In fact, our genetic makeup can influence how susceptible we are to addiction. However, it's important to remember that just because someone is genetically susceptible to addiction, that doesn't necessarily mean that he or she will become an addict. It just means that he or she is at risk.

- Which genes make someone more susceptible to addiction, and how can we find those genes? Finding the offending genes turns out to be extremely difficult. Our genetic material is stored in 23 pairs of chromosomes in the nucleus of cells. Each chromosome is a molecule of DNA, which is wrapped tightly into a sequence of bundles, and each of those DNA molecules is long. In fact, if you uncoiled the DNA in just one of your cells it would be about 6 feet long.

- The rungs on the ladder of DNA are made of molecules called nucleotide bases that are arranged in pairs. There's a lot of genetic information encoded in your 6 feet of DNA. There are often over 100 million rungs on the ladder in just one chromosome. And with 23 pairs of chromosomes, there are well over 3 billion rungs in total in each cell.

- Genes are small sections of each of these ladders, ranging in length from a few hundred nucleotide base rungs to well over a million. We all have over 20,000 genes, and each of them encodes the information needed to make a few of the hundreds of thousands of proteins that do a lot of the biological work in your body. And exactly which proteins get made is what makes you who you are: Your height, your natural hair and eye color, your skin color, and even your intelligence and personality are significantly affected by the proteins encoded by your genes.

- The two chromosomes in each pair contain the same genes in exactly the same places, but they might be different versions of those genes. The version of a gene in one chromosome comes from your mother, and the version of the gene in the paired chromosome comes from your father. Each version of a gene is called an allele.

- You might inherit one allele of a gene from your mother that gives you a lot of freckles, but the same gene from your father on the other chromosome might be an allele that is not associated with freckles. Whether you have a lot of freckles or not would then depend on whether one of the versions is dominant.

- So, we inherit two versions of each gene from our parents, and apparently one or more of these genes can influence our susceptibility to addiction. In particular, some gene variants, or alleles, might increase susceptibility while others might decrease risk. But which genes are these, and how can we find them on this 6-foot-long, 3-billion-rung ladder of DNA?

- Finding genes can be very difficult. Geneticists therefore often try to narrow down the search using a technique called linkage analysis. The key idea behind linkage analysis is that geneticists know that if one part of the DNA ladder gets passed down to a child, then nearby parts are also likely to get passed down from that same ladder. That is, nearby parts of a DNA ladder are likely to be linked and passed down together.

- How can we use this fact about linkage to narrow down the search for genes related to an addiction? We can start with a whole bunch of genetic markers whose location we already know. Think of choosing 400 rungs of the DNA ladders that are spread out over all the chromosomes. Suppose that one of those markers is linked with an addiction gene, meaning that the two almost always get inherited together. Then, we can infer that the addiction gene we're looking for must be close to that marker.

- To do this, geneticists analyze DNA samples from people in large, extended families that contain many addicts. Then, they look for genetic markers that get inherited with the addiction. When they find one, they can narrow down the search to the area around the linked genetic marker. Once they've found a promising area on a specific chromosome, geneticists will then often perform what are called association studies in order to try to identify the specific gene in that region that is associated with the addiction.

- The first step is to identify parts of the DNA that are in the target region and that differ in different individuals. It turns out that the vast majority of the rungs on the human DNA ladder are the same in everyone. In fact, if you compared the DNA of any two normal humans, you would find that over 99 percent of the rungs are the same.

- So, the rungs that differ account for a lot of the variability we see among different human beings. Those rungs that vary are called polymorphisms. Furthermore, because the rungs are made of nucleotide bases, the individual rungs that differ across different people are typically called single nucleotide polymorphisms (SNPs), which play a big role in genetic association studies.

- Association studies of addiction analyze genetic data from thousands of people, some of whom are addicts and some of whom are not. And they look at what form of a target SNP each person has. If a particular form of an SNP occurs significantly more frequently in the addicts than it does in the nonaddicts, then that SNP is said to be associated with the addiction, and a gene near that SNP is likely involved.

- In recent years, techniques have been developed that make it possible to analyze huge numbers of SNPs simultaneously. In fact, geneticists can now analyze SNPs covering the entire genome—that is, all the DNA in all the chromosomes. This kind of genome-wide association study makes it possible to find new genes that might contribute to addiction even without a prior linkage analysis.

- By now, dozens of linkage and association studies have been done to investigate the genetics of addiction and to identify genes that might influence susceptibility. The results of these studies have shown two general things. First, there is no single addiction gene. Second, the same genes contribute to many different addictions.

- So, there may actually be a scientific basis to the idea of an addictive personality—that is, of a person who is at risk of getting hooked on any kind of addictive substance or behavior. These findings may also explain why so many

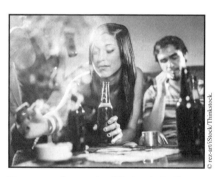

There may be a scientific basis to the idea of an addictive personality.

addicts have multiple addictions—for example, to both alcohol and nicotine. And they may shed light on why some people get addicted to specific behaviors, such as gambling or video games, that don't even involve consuming an addictive substance.

- Why should geneticists bother to figure out where a gene is? Geneticists aren't typically interested in figuring out the location of a gene as an end in itself. Once they've figured out where a gene is, then, and only then, they can begin to study what it does. And understanding what a gene does can provide insight as to why some people are more susceptible to addiction than others.

Genetic Engineering to Study Addiction

- How can we figure out what a gene does? Geneticists often turn to mice to answer this question, as well. In fact, they often genetically engineer mice to answer this question. Genetic engineering refers to intentionally changing or engineering some aspect of the DNA of an organism.

- One very powerful technique is knocking out the operation of a particular gene in a set of mice and then observing their behavior compared with normal mice. Differences in the behavior of these so-called knockout mice can often shed light on the function of the target gene.

- One particularly powerful example comes from studying the genetics of nicotine addiction and the role of a chemical called acetylcholine, which is a neurotransmitter that some brain cells use to communicate with each other. When a brain cell releases acetylcholine, the acetylcholine can attach to special molecules called acetylcholine receptors on other brain cells, which could lead those cells to become active.

- Nicotine can also attach to these receptors and can therefore mimic the effects of acetylcholine. In fact, because these receptors respond to nicotine, they're typically called nicotinic acetylcholine receptors. These receptors, like most complex biological structures, are made up of proteins, which are made by genes. And it turns out that some of the genes that linkage and association studies found were associated with addiction to cigarettes were actually genes that encoded the proteins that make up nicotinic acetylcholine receptors.

- This led geneticists to a specific hypothesis: Maybe some versions of these genes make the receptors more responsive to nicotine and therefore increase susceptibility to nicotine addiction, while other versions of these genes make the receptors less responsive and decrease susceptibility.

- To test this idea, they genetically engineered mice that lacked these genes entirely. They found that normal mice will self-administer nicotine and show many of the behavioral symptoms of nicotine addiction, but these genetically engineered mice did not.

- Recall that all addictive substances lead to increased levels of dopamine in the limbic system, which may be associated with wanting or craving. Nicotine does the same thing—or at least it does in normal mice. However, the genetically engineered mice did not show an increase in dopamine when nicotine was administered. It's as if the genetically engineered mice were no longer susceptible to nicotine addiction.

- Many other knockout studies of addiction have been performed, and they've taught us a lot about how different genes contribute to addiction. For example, knocking out one gene produces mice that are less sensitive to painkillers, such as morphine, compared with normal mice. Knocking out another gene leads to mice that are unusually attracted to cocaine. Still other knockout mice are less likely to develop morphine dependence. And others are more sensitive to the effects of alcohol.

- These kinds of findings are particularly exciting because they offer the hope of new and better treatments for addiction. Every time a gene is identified that contributes to addiction, that gene becomes a potential target for a biologically based treatment. For example, once we understand how a genetic variant increases addiction risk, we could potentially design treatments to counteract those effects. Likewise, if a genetic variant is found that is protective and decreases risk, we could design treatments that mimic and strengthen that effect.

- Furthermore, treatments could be tailored to the specific genetic profile of a particular individual. For example, different people might be susceptible to alcohol addiction for very different reasons. The most effective treatment could be different for these different people. By analyzing their genetic profile, physicians in the future might be able to design a treatment program that is personalized specifically for them.

Suggested Reading

Crabbe, "Genetic Contributions to Addiction."

Genetic Science Learning Center, The University of Utah, "The New Science of Addiction."

Li and Burmeister, "New Insights into the Genetics of Addiction."

Ridley, *The Agile Gene*.

Questions to Consider

1. What is some of the evidence that certain people are innately more susceptible to addiction than others?

2. How do geneticists go about finding genes that contribute to addiction susceptibility?

3. Can you reconcile the neural and genetic findings on addiction with the idea that drug users have free will?

Your Brain on Drugs
Lecture 5

In this lecture, you will learn about how drugs affect the brain. First, you will learn about the psychological effects of psychoactive drugs. How can chemicals make us feel relaxed, or elevate our mood, or increase our focus? Second, what determines the strength of a drug's effects? Finally, you will learn about how we can become dependent on drugs. In general, this lecture will give you a basic understanding of how psychoactive drugs work and produce their effects.

The Psychological Effects of Psychoactive Drugs

- Neurons typically communicate using chemicals called neurotransmitters, examples of which are dopamine, serotonin, and acetylcholine. This communication takes place in the very small spaces, called synapses, between neurons.

- When a brain cell is activated, it generates an electrical potential that travels down the neuron to the synapses between it and neighboring neurons. When the electrical potential reaches the synapses, it causes the cell to release a bunch of neurotransmitter molecules. These molecules then move across the synapses, and they may come into contact with neighboring neurons, perhaps exciting them and causing them to fire, too. In this way, a neural signal can travel from neuron to neuron through a brain circuit.

- Neurotransmitters cause a neighboring neuron to fire by binding to receptor molecules on the surface of the next neuron. Receptors are like small machines in the cell. When they're turned on, they can make the neuron more likely to fire. If enough receptors are turned on at the same time, that can trigger the neuron to become active and release its own neurotransmitters in downstream synapses. Some receptors are also inhibitory, and if they get turned on, they actually try to prevent the neuron from firing.

- When a neurotransmitter binds to a receptor, it's like a key being slid into a machine and turning it on. And just as a key only fits certain locks, a neurotransmitter only fits certain receptors, and it will only bind to them. Dopamine binds to dopamine receptors, serotonin binds to serotonin receptors, and so on.

- How do psychoactive drugs produce psychological effects? One way they do so is by binding to and turning on the same receptors that natural neurotransmitters do. So, in a very real sense, psychoactive drugs imitate natural brain chemicals.

- But why do they produce different effects than the natural neurotransmitters themselves? One reason is that psychoactive drugs may activate the receptors more or less strongly than the natural neurotransmitters do. Even though the receptors are doing what they normally do, the level of activity may be abnormal, and that can lead to observable psychological effects.

The Strength of a Drug's Effects
- What determines the strength of a drug's psychological effects? One very important factor is how much of the drug actually gets to the brain—for example, how much of the drug gets into the bloodstream, how much is metabolized and converted to something else, and so on. There's an entire field called pharmacokinetics devoted to these issues.

- What happens after the drug reaches the brain, and how can that affect a drug's strength? The law of mass action is a very general chemical principle, but in this context, it basically means that the more molecules there are in a synapse, the more receptors will be active.

- When a neurotransmitter or a psychoactive drug binds to a receptor, it doesn't stay there forever. Rather, most molecules bind reversibly—that is, they bind for an instant; turn on the receptor; and then unbind, or dissociate, from the receptor, turning the receptor off. Then, another neurotransmitter molecule might come along and bind to that receptor and turn it on for a moment again, before it, too, dissociates. And this same process happens over and over again. This process is random, or stochastic.

- If there are many neurotransmitter molecules, or drug molecules, in the synapse, then there's a high probability that one of them will run into a receptor and turn it on. And even after that molecule dissociates from the receptor, another molecule is likely to run into that receptor and turn it on right away.

- The more neurotransmitter, or drug, molecules you have in the synapse, the more receptors will be turned on. That's also why larger drug doses have larger effects. Larger doses mean more drug molecules in the synapses, and the more molecules in the synapses, the larger the effect.

- But that's only true up to a point. As you add more and more of the drug, you eventually reach a point where virtually all the receptors are bound by drug molecules: As soon as one molecule dissociates from a receptor, there's another molecule there to immediately take its place. At that point, adding more of the drug can no longer increase the drug's effect, because all the receptors are already active all the time.

- This relationship between the dose of a drug and the response to the drug can be represented graphically in what's called a dose-response curve. The overall dose-response curve is S-shaped, or what's sometimes called a sigmoid curve.

- Why do some drugs have stronger effects than others? One key difference lies in what's called the affinity of the drug for the receptors. Recall the lock-and-key analogy. Imagine a key that is sticky and that you have to jiggle to get out of the lock, versus a key that slides in and out very easily. The sticky key has high affinity: It tends to stay in the lock, and it's more difficult to get it out.

- Likewise, a drug that has high affinity for a receptor tends to bind strongly and is more difficult to get out. It therefore doesn't dissociate as quickly but, rather, stays bound to the receptors longer and keeps them active. On the other hand, a molecule that has low affinity is like a key that slides in and out of the lock very easily: It may bind to a receptor, but it's a loose fit, so it dissociates very quickly.

- A low dose of a high-affinity drug will lead to a larger response than a low dose of a low-affinity drug. Put another way, drugs with high affinity are more potent than drugs with low affinity. Here, potency refers to the amount of drug you need to get a specific level of response.

- Surprisingly, the affinity of a drug does not actually determine its maximum possible effect, or what is often called a drug's efficacy. So, then, what does determine the efficacy of a drug? For example, why is the maximum possible level of pain relief so much higher for morphine than it is for aspirin?

- One reason two drugs could have different efficacies is because they act in different ways. For example, if two drugs bind to different types of receptors, and one of those receptors is more related to pain relief than the other one, then it wouldn't be surprising if the drugs differ in how much pain relief they can provide.

- But even if two drugs bind to the same type of receptor, they could still have different efficacies if they drive the receptors to different degrees. The degree to which a molecule drives a receptor is referred as its intrinsic activity, and it can differ for different molecules. And differences in intrinsic activity lead to differences in the maximum effect that a drug can have.

- A drug with high intrinsic activity produces a strong response from the receptor, whereas a drug with low intrinsic activity produces a weak response, even though it's bound to the same receptor. Those two drugs could produce significantly different responses even if all the receptors are continuously bound, so the efficacy, or maximum possible effect, for the two drugs would be quite different.

- Why do some drugs have stronger psychological effects than others? One important reason is because different drugs differ in their affinity and in the amount of intrinsic activity that they produce. Drugs with higher affinity are more potent, meaning that you need less of the drug to produce an effect. And drugs that produce higher intrinsic activity have higher efficacy, meaning that they produce a larger maximum effect.

- Understanding how drugs affect the brain can also provide some insight into some of the pharmacological treatments that are used to treat drug overdose. To understand how these medicines work, it's helpful to distinguish between agonists and antagonists. An agonist is a molecule that binds to a receptor and produces high intrinsic activity—that is, it drives the receptor strongly. Antagonists, on the other hand, bind to the same receptors, but they produce no intrinsic activity.

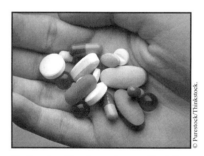

- Antagonists produce their effects by blocking the action of an agonist, whether the agonist is a natural neurotransmitter or a drug. Antagonists, as well as chemicals that serve as partial agonists, are used in treating drug addicts.

Understanding how drugs affect the brain can provide insight into some of the pharmacological treatments that are used to treat drug overdose.

Drug Dependency

- How can someone become dependent on a drug? And, specifically, what are some of the neural mechanisms underlying the symptoms of tolerance and withdrawal? After repeated drug use, people often need more of the drug to get the same effect. That is, they become tolerant to the effects of the drug. In fact, chronic drug users often report not feeling the same high as they used to but that they still need to take their drug just to feel normal again.

- What's happening is that the body has begun to compensate for the presence of the drug. That is, the body has gotten used to the drug, and it's trying to compensate for this abnormal chemical by adapting in specific ways. Essentially, it's the body's attempt to return to normal functioning despite the drug.

- The body can do this in many ways, and some of these changes happen outside the brain. For example, chronic alcoholics produce more of the enzyme that breaks down alcohol than nonalcoholics do. So, less alcohol will get into the blood and brain than in nonalcoholics. As a result, alcoholics become tolerant to alcohol, and they need to drink more to have the same effect.

- But there are also changes that are occurring within the brain itself. In particular, over time, the brain will often reduce the number of receptors that the drug is binding to. This is called receptor downregulation. Essentially, the body is expecting large quantities of the drug, and in order to reduce the effect of that drug, it reduces the number of receptors that respond to it.

- The body is trying to maintain a stable level of receptor activity by reducing the number of receptors. Naturally, if there are fewer receptors, then the same amount of drug will produce a smaller effect. So, tolerance develops.

- Receptor downregulation can also help explain why people experience withdrawal or abstinence syndrome. Once someone gets used to taking a drug and the number of receptors that the drug binds to has been reduced, when the drug is removed, he or she tends to experience symptoms that are the opposite of those produced by the drug itself.

- In a sense, withdrawal symptoms are the mirror image of the effects that the drug itself produces. The body has gotten used to a large quantity of the drug in the system and has compensated by downregulating receptors. When the drug is removed, the few remaining receptors are not being activated as much as they previously were, so you get the opposite effects of the drug itself.

- When we talk about dependence on a drug, one of the things we mean is that tolerance has developed. That is, there have been some physical changes in the body that have led to tolerance to the presence of the drug, and now quitting the drug will result in withdrawal symptoms. These could be physical symptoms or psychological symptoms.

Suggested Reading

Kranzier, Ciraulo, and Zindel, eds., *Clinical Manual of Addiction Psychopharmacology*.

Meyer and Quenzer, *Psychopharmacology*.

Nestler, Hyman, and Malenka, *Molecular Neuropharmacology*.

Snyder, *Drugs and the Brain*.

Valenstein, *The War of the Soups and the Sparks*.

Questions to Consider

1. How can a lock-and-key analogy be used to explain how psychoactive drugs have their effects?

2. What is the difference between a drug's potency and its efficacy, and what factors influence each?

3. How can the same dose of a drug produce less and less of an effect over time?

Why We Crave Coffee and Cigarettes
Lecture 6

This lecture is about two of the most widely used psychoactive drugs in the world: caffeine and nicotine. They are both legal and widely available, and billions of people use them on a daily basis. In this lecture, you will dive into the details of these two drugs of abuse to learn how each works at a neural level. In addition to learning what's going on in the brain, you will learn about the latest treatments that are available.

Caffeine

- Caffeine is by far the most-used psychoactive drug in the world. Eighty to ninety percent of Americans drink coffee or other caffeinated drinks every day. A typical adult consumes 200 to 400 milligrams of caffeine every day on average. But is the regular consumption of caffeine really a problem?

- Except in severe cases, consuming caffeine on a regular basis doesn't pose a significant health risk. In fact, moderate caffeine use has actually been associated with a number of health benefits, including reduced risk of Parkinson's disease and type 2 diabetes. Caffeine also has a number of behavioral benefits, including increased alertness and improved concentration.

- But despite these positive effects, caffeine is not a vitamin. It's a mild psychoactive drug that works in ways that are similar to other more dangerous psychoactive drugs. And regular use of caffeine can and does lead to physical dependence and the associated symptoms of tolerance and withdrawal, just like regular use of other drugs does.

- What does caffeine do to the brain? Caffeine is an adenosine receptor antagonist, which means that it binds to the same receptors as the brain chemical adenosine, but it doesn't turn on the receptor. It just prevents the adenosine from turning on the receptors.

- Adenosine is an inhibitory brain chemical, meaning that it tends to reduce neural activity. Furthermore, adenosine levels in the brain continuously rise when we're awake, and then they fall back down when we sleep. Many scientists therefore believe that adenosine serves an important role in our sleep-wake cycle.

- Caffeine blocks the effect of adenosine and therefore helps us stay awake even if it's past our normal bedtime. Essentially, the caffeine fools the brain into thinking that it hasn't been awake for as long as it has. Consistent with this interpretation, knockout mice that lack adenosine receptors don't show the normal stimulating effects of caffeine.

- While there are quite a few similarities between caffeine and other more dangerous psychoactive drugs, there are also some significant differences between caffeine and these other drugs. One very important difference involves the level of stimulation of the reward circuit.

- Drugs of abuse significantly overstimulate the reward circuit, and repeated overstimulation can produce cravings so strong that they lead to unhealthy and even life-threatening behavior. That's the kind of positive reinforcement that is typically associated with real addiction.

- In contrast, caffeine use doesn't produce that same kind of positive reinforcement. Studies have found that caffeine is only weakly reinforcing; animals are not obsessed with getting caffeine in the same way they are with more dangerous drugs.

- In fact, scientists believe that people often consume caffeine just to avoid the negative withdrawal symptoms of fatigue and irritability, not because it stimulates the brain's reward circuit. That's more of a negative reinforcement situation, in which continued drug use is motivated by a desire to avoid unpleasant effects. Positive reinforcement is probably a better model of addiction for serious drugs than is negative reinforcement. Another important difference between caffeine and other addictive drugs is that chronic caffeine use doesn't typically lead to the severe negative consequences.

- For these reasons, caffeine is not considered to be a drug of abuse. Repeated use can, and actually does, lead to changes in the brain and, ultimately, to physical dependence. But that use doesn't typically lead to significant negative consequences or distress. On the contrary, for most people, not drinking their coffee would lead to negative consequences and distress.

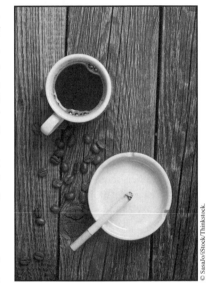

Nicotine

- Nicotine is another very commonly used drug. This psychoactive drug is also legal and also has stimulating effects that bear

Caffeine and nicotine are two of the most widely used psychoactive drugs.

a resemblance to caffeine's effects. But unlike caffeine, nicotine is one of the most addictive substances in the world, and taking it can have life-threatening consequences.

- Nicotine is actually a naturally produced insecticide. Purified nicotine was used as an insecticide by farmers for a number of years, but they stopped using it because it was too toxic to humans. In fact, 60 milligrams of nicotine is all it takes to kill an adult human being. Yet this toxic chemical is also extremely addictive at low doses, as the enormous number of smokers demonstrates.

- Roughly one-third of the world's adult population smokes tobacco on a regular basis, and roughly 80 percent of them started before they turned 18. The same thing is true in rats. Specifically, if rats start self-administering nicotine during adolescence, then they self-administer significantly more than rats that start administering nicotine in adulthood.

- Tobacco smoke contains thousands of chemicals other than nicotine, and the health consequences of inhaling those chemicals on a regular basis are disastrous. For example, cigarette smoke contains more than 50 chemicals that are known to cause cancer. Cigarette smoke also contains tar, a collection of solid particles that forms a sticky brown residue on smokers' teeth, fingers, and lungs. Tar is also carcinogenic.

- Regularly inhaling these chemicals is very bad for you. In fact, smoking-related illnesses are estimated to kill more than 5 million people every year. In particular, smoking is estimated to be responsible for 80 to 90 percent of lung cancer deaths.

- And for every person who dies, there are approximately 20 other smokers who suffer from at least one serious illness associated with smoking, such as heart disease or stroke. The life expectancy of smokers is more than 10 years shorter than nonsmokers.

- Most smokers don't want to smoke, but they're hooked on the nicotine. Approximately 70 to 75 percent of smokers say they'd like to quit, and 40 percent of regular smokers try to quit every year. But it's a very tough habit to kick. In fact, fewer than 10 percent of quit attempts end up succeeding in the long term. That's comparable to the quit rate for heroin.

- The behavioral effects of nicotine are relatively mild and are similar to those of caffeine. Low doses of nicotine increase arousal and can actually improve concentration and enhance performance in attention-demanding tasks, even in nonsmokers. But nicotine can also lead to tension and light-headedness. And higher doses can produce nausea, sweating, and dizziness.

- Chronic smokers actually become tolerant to many of these effects and often find smoking to be relaxing rather than arousing. They also exhibit withdrawal symptoms when their nicotine levels drop: They'll become irritable and stressed and report difficulty concentrating. Many scientists believe that the relaxing effect of cigarettes in smokers may simply reflect relief from these negative withdrawal symptoms.

- Like caffeine and other psychoactive drugs, nicotine works by binding to receptors used by a normal brain chemical. And in this case, the normal brain chemical is the neurotransmitter acetylcholine, which is the neurotransmitter that is used to tell our muscles to contract and is also associated with arousal, vigilance, and paying attention. It also plays an important role in the sleep-wake cycle.

- Nicotine is an agonist for a class of acetylcholine receptors. Recall that an agonist is a chemical that binds to a receptor and strongly activates it. Nicotine strongly activates acetylcholine receptors. In fact, the receptors that it activates have actually been named after nicotine: nicotinic acetylcholine receptors. A number of studies have now demonstrated that the way nicotine produces its effects is by binding to these nicotinic acetylcholine receptors.

- Nicotine is binding to the same receptors as acetylcholine and putting them in overdrive. And because acetylcholine is associated with alertness and vigilance, so is nicotine. But why is nicotine so addictive? To answer that question, we need to return to the brain's reward circuit. Recall that one very important region in the brain's reward circuit is the ventral tegmental area (VTA). Neurons in the VTA communicate using the neurotransmitter dopamine, referred to as the addiction molecule of the brain. More dopamine is associated with more incentive salience, or more wanting or craving.

- Nicotine binds to the acetylcholine receptors on the VTA dopamine neurons and puts them into overdrive, overstimulating the reward circuit. The VTA dopamine neurons therefore fire a lot, and they release unusually large quantities of dopamine. This large dopamine release has two important consequences that contribute to addiction: It triggers wanting or craving, and it signals the need for more learning and the strengthening of neural pathways.

- Chronic smoking leads to the repeated release of high levels of dopamine by activation of the nicotinic acetylcholine receptors on the VTA neurons. Over time, that dopamine signal backs up to the environmental cues that are associated with smoking—for example, a pack of cigarettes, a book of matches, the smell of smoke, the inside of a bar, and so on.

- Eventually, any and all of these environmental stimuli become triggers that will lead to dopamine release themselves. And the dopamine is what produces the strong craving, which leads to more smoking. The longer this cycle repeats, the stronger the associations become. Pretty soon, it's virtually impossible to resist the urge to smoke, and an addiction is born.

- Another reason smoking is so addictive is that it's an extremely efficient method for delivering nicotine to the brain. Ingesting low doses of nicotine isn't particularly addictive. Even intravenous administration of nicotine is less addictive than smoking, because smoking gets the nicotine to the brain extremely quickly. In fact, nicotine reaches the brain about seven seconds after a puff on a cigarette, and that fast action appears to contribute to its addictiveness.

Treatment Options for Smokers
- There are a number of treatment options that have been scientifically proven to help motivated smokers kick the habit. One very common approach is called nicotine replacement therapy, which involves providing low-dose nicotine without smoking and then gradually decreasing the dose over time until the smoker has kicked the nicotine habit entirely.

- There are now five FDA-approved approaches to nicotine replacement therapy: the nicotine patch, nicotine gum, nicotine lozenges, nicotine nasal spray, and the nicotine inhaler. Both the nasal spray and the inhaler deliver nicotine quickly and can be used as needed to control urges. But they both also require a prescription. On the other hand, nicotine gum, lozenges, and patches are all now available over the counter without a prescription.

- Studies find that smokers receiving nicotine replacement are roughly twice as likely to quit as smokers in control groups. So, nicotine replacement does seem to help. The bad news is that most people still don't manage to quit.

- Another product that's become quite popular is the electronic cigarette, or e-cigarette, but it's controversial. E-cigarettes are similar to nicotine inhalers. When the user takes a drag, the e-cigarette creates a vapor containing nicotine that is inhaled. E-cigarettes haven't undergone the same rigorous testing as standard nicotine replacement therapies and haven't been approved by the FDA as a smoking cessation treatment. There is also concern that they might be tempting to nonsmokers, especially children, because they're easier to get and often include flavors that might appeal to children.

- Behavioral therapy attempts to break the strong associations between smoking and a variety of environmental triggers that smokers have. Smokers in behavioral therapy often work on recognizing the triggers that are the most strongly associated with smoking for them. Then, they work on strategies for avoiding those triggers or coping with them when they do encounter them.

- Combining behavioral therapy with nicotine replacement therapy is significantly more effective than either method alone. Dealing with both the physical and psychological side of the addiction simultaneously can really help.

Suggested Reading

Luttinger and Dicum, *The Coffee Book*.

Mayo Clinic, "Nicotine Dependence."

National Cancer Institute, "Smokefree.Gov."

————, "Tobacco Statistics."

Nehlig, "Are We Dependent upon Coffee and Caffeine?"

Proctor, *Golden Holocaust*.

Questions to Consider

1. Why is nicotine dependence considered an addiction while caffeine dependence isn't?

2. What does nicotine do in the brain, and how does it produce addiction?

3. What are some of approaches being used to help smokers quit?

Alcohol—Social Lubricant or Drug of Abuse?
Lecture 7

Our society often treats alcohol as a relatively harmless social lubricant rather than as a drug of abuse. But is it really different than other addictive drugs? In this lecture, you will learn how alcohol affects the human body and how it is similar to the way that other addictive drugs affect the body. You also will learn about the ways in which alcohol is different from other drugs of abuse. Finally, you will learn about various treatment options for alcoholism.

How Does Alcohol Affect the Brain?

- Neurons in the brain typically communicate using special chemicals called neurotransmitters. One neuron releases a bunch of neurotransmitter molecules, and these molecules bind to receptors on neighboring neurons, potentially activating those receptors and producing specific biological effects.

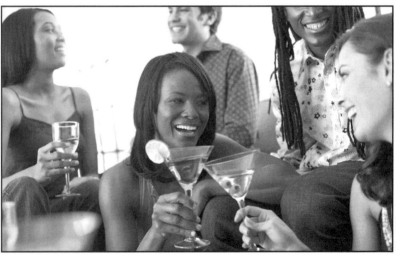

© Fuse/Thinkstock.

Our society treats alcohol as a relatively harmless social lubricant, though its effects on the body are similar to those of other addictive drugs.

- Drugs of abuse typically bind to the same receptors as natural neurotransmitters but then produce abnormal levels of activity in those receptors. And that abnormal activity is what makes the drugs psychoactive, making the user experience particular feelings, such as euphoria, excitement, or contentment.

- Alcohol also binds to natural receptors and produces abnormal receptor activity. In fact, alcohol affects receptors for multiple neurotransmitters, and two of the most important are called glutamate and GABA.

- Glutamate is the major excitatory neurotransmitter in the brain. It's the chemical that many neurons use to try to make neighboring neurons fire. Glutamate has a few different receptors, but the one that's most influenced by alcohol is the NMDA receptor. These receptors have been found to play a major role in learning and memory.

- Alcohol binds to NMDA receptors and makes them less active. NMDA receptors have multiple binding sites, and alcohol binds to a different site on the receptor than glutamate. When alcohol binds, it actually changes the receptor and makes it less responsive to glutamate. This is called allosteric modulation. The alcohol is modulating the effects of glutamate by binding to a different site on the NMDA receptors.

- Alcohol reduces the effects that glutamate normally has; glutamate normally excites neurons and makes them fire. By inhibiting or antagonizing glutamate, alcohol suppresses neural activity in the brain. And that's why it produces a sedative and hypnotic effect. Also, the fact that NMDA receptors play an important role in learning and memory may explain why large doses of alcohol can produce blackouts and amnesia.

- The other major neurotransmitter that alcohol affects is GABA. While glutamate is the brain's major excitatory neurotransmitter, GABA is its major inhibitory neurotransmitter. When GABA receptors on a neuron are activated, they try to prevent the neuron from firing. So, increasing the activity of GABA actually suppresses neural activity.

- Scientists have not yet found a particular site on the GABA receptors where alcohol binds. Nevertheless, most scientists still believe that alcohol is again acting as an allosteric modulator, but this time making GABA receptors more responsive to GABA and therefore suppressing neural activity. And the reason they believe this is because the effects of alcohol are so similar to drugs that do bind to GABA receptors—in particular, barbiturate drugs.

Alcohol versus Drugs of Abuse
- Alcohol shares at least one important characteristic with drugs of abuse: They both bind to natural receptors in the brain and lead to abnormal levels of activity. A second characteristic of drugs of abuse is that repeated use can lead to compensatory changes in the body that produce physical dependence, which is characterized by tolerance to the drug's effects and withdrawal symptoms when the drug is stopped.

- Chronic alcohol use produces similar compensatory changes and physical dependence. People who drink a lot for an extended period of time will typically become less sensitive to alcohol's effects over time. They develop a tolerance for alcohol. There are actually a number of changes that happen in the body that contribute to alcohol tolerance, including changes in the digestive system that allow a person to break down alcohol faster than they could originally, resulting in having to drink more to have the same effect.

- Compensatory changes also occur in the brain. In particular, there's evidence for an upregulation of NMDA receptors and a downregulation of GABA receptors in the brains of heavy drinkers. Recall that alcohol binds to NMDA receptors and inhibits the activity of glutamate. If you continuously and chronically use alcohol, the brain will try to compensate for that by producing more NMDA receptors. That's upregulation. Conversely, chronic alcohol use leads to downregulation of GABA receptors. In this case, the brain is compensating for the overstimulation of these GABA receptors by producing fewer of those receptors.

- And these compensatory changes contribute to alcohol tolerance. In most people, alcohol produces sedative and hypnotic effects because of the way it inhibits neural processing. But the brain of the chronic alcohol drinker has reduced its ability to produce inhibition. Consequently, alcoholics won't experience the same amount of sedation; they become tolerant to the effects of alcohol, a clear sign of physical dependence.

- Heavy drinkers who quit experience withdrawal symptoms that are worse than withdrawal symptoms from most drugs of abuse. In fact, withdrawal from alcohol can be quite dangerous, even fatal. Standard symptoms of alcohol withdrawal include tremors and shakes, high anxiety, high blood pressure, increased heart rate, sweating, and nausea. In severe cases, alcoholics in withdrawal may experience delirium tremens. It's therefore important for a heavy drinker who wants to quit to do so under a doctor's supervision.

- What's causing these severe withdrawal symptoms? If alcohol is discontinued after the upregulation and downregulation of brain receptors, then there are more NMDA receptors than normal, but now the alcohol isn't there to inhibit the excitatory actions of glutamate. So, you get abnormally high levels of neural activity. Worse yet, the downregulation of GABA receptors means that there are fewer of them to inhibit neural processing and keep it in check.

- The end result is substantial overstimulation when alcohol is stopped. And it's that overstimulation that is thought to give rise to the seizures and anxiety that are associated with alcohol withdrawal. The alcoholic is now physically dependent on alcohol and needs to drink just to feel normal.

- A third characteristic of drugs of abuse is their addictiveness. Alcohol is certainly addictive. In fact, the World Health Organization estimated that there are approximately 140 million people addicted to alcohol worldwide, making alcohol the single most-abused substance on the planet. But are the mechanisms underlying alcohol addiction similar to the mechanisms underlying addiction to drugs of abuse?

- Drugs of abuse overstimulate the brain's reward circuit. They tend to excite or activate the nucleus accumbens, which is associated with feelings of pleasure. They also tend to lead to a release of dopamine by neurons in the ventral tegmental area (VTA). And that dopamine release is associated with craving or wanting. That dopamine release will back up to cues that are associated with the drug taking. So, now when the drug user encounters those cues, dopamine is released and they may experience strong craving to use the drug.

- These same mechanisms are at work in the brains of alcoholics. Consider the brain's pleasure center, the nucleus accumbens. Drugs that block the response of the nucleus accumbens also reduce the desire to drink alcohol. Research has found that alcohol must be activating the nucleus accumbens and producing a reward response just like drugs of abuse do.

- In addition, like drugs of abuse, alcohol has also been shown to lead to increased dopamine release in the reward circuit. Alcoholics also have very strong triggers associated with alcohol use, just like drug addicts have triggers associated with drug use.

- Furthermore, just like other addictions, there is very good evidence for genetic susceptibility to alcohol addiction; apparently, your genetic makeup can influence your desire to drink.

- Despite the similarities that alcohol shares with drugs of abuse, alcohol is different from drugs of abuse on other grounds. For example, alcohol is legal while some other drugs are not. It's also much more socially acceptable than so-called harder drugs. More importantly, there's some evidence that although alcohol is addictive, it's not as addictive as cocaine or heroin—or nicotine, for that matter.

- Chronic alcohol use is also associated with a number of significant negative consequences, just like the chronic use of other drugs. Excessive drinking, and drinking at inappropriate times, is associated with some very significant health risks. For example, long-term, heavy drinking can lead to cirrhosis of the liver. It can also cause brain damage and shrinkage of the cerebral cortex. And, of course, drinking and driving can have fatal consequences. Heavy alcohol use can even lead to malnutrition.

Treatment Options for Alcoholism

- The first step in treating an addiction to alcohol is typically detoxification, which means weaning the person off of alcohol for a long enough period of time that his or her physical dependence has subsided and he or she isn't experiencing severe withdrawal symptoms anymore. Detoxification often involves providing a substitute for alcohol that can mimic some of its inhibitory effects, in order to prevent the severe overstimulation that typically occurs during alcohol withdrawal.

- In particular, physicians will often prescribe benzodiazepines, such as Valium, during detoxification. Benzodiazepines activate the inhibitory GABA receptors like alcohol does, so taking them when you're quitting alcohol helps to prevent the dangerous symptoms, such as seizures and delirium tremens, that are associated with alcohol withdrawal.

- After detoxification, the next step is often some kind of psychosocial rehabilitation. This could be individual or group therapy, or it could be a self-help group like Alcoholics Anonymous, Rational Recovery, or the Community Reinforcement Approach.

- All of these psychosocial methods seem to help, in the sense that people who participate are more likely to quit drinking than people who don't. However, they don't work for everyone. In fact, roughly 40 to 70 percent of people in the programs are drinking again after one year. Nevertheless, it's often helpful to see failures as learning opportunities and as normal steps in the road to complete abstinence.

- There are also some pharmacological interventions that have proven to help drinkers quit. One common approach is a drug called disulfiram, which inhibits one of the enzymes that breaks down alcohol. By inhibiting this enzyme, people aren't able to break down alcohol as efficiently as they normally do. As a result, they have a very unpleasant reaction to alcohol, such as intense, unpleasant hangover-like symptoms.

- The hope is that these symptoms will make drinking aversive, and people will feel less of an urge to drink. One problem with this approach is that you have to be very determined to quit drinking for it to work. Otherwise, you'll simply stop taking the drug.

- A second pharmacological approach is to try to eliminate the rewarding effects of alcohol. Alcohol activates the nucleus accumbens, the brain's pleasure center. A drug called naltrexone tries to help alcoholics quit by inhibiting that pleasure response. Reducing the pleasure associated with drinking can help alcoholics quit, especially when naltrexone is combined with behavioral therapy. In fact, quit rates double after three months of such a treatment combination.

- A third medication that has proven somewhat effective in helping alcoholics is called acamprosate. This medication can reduce the unpleasant side effects of alcohol withdrawal and hopefully help the recovering alcoholic stay abstinent.

Suggested Reading

Blum, *Alcohol and the Addictive Brain*.

Gately, *Drink*.

Ketcham, Asbury, Schulstad, and Ciaramicoli, *Beyond the Influence*.

Questions to Consider

1. What are the neural mechanisms that underlie alcohol's psychological effects?

2. Why should a chronic alcoholic not try to quit cold turkey without medical supervision?

3. Do you think that alcohol should be considered a drug of abuse?

The Science of Marijuana
Lecture 8

S ome people see marijuana as a dangerous, addictive drug, and they often think of medical marijuana as a loophole that drug dealers and addicts use to skirt the law. Other people see marijuana as a relatively harmless drug and one that has some beneficial properties that could help patients suffering from a number of illnesses. What does science have to say about marijuana? What does marijuana do to the brain, and what kinds of effects does it have? Does it have any demonstrated medical benefits? How addictive is it? These are the kinds of questions that will be addressed in this lecture.

Marijuana and the Brain

- Marijuana comes from the hemp plant, *Cannabis sativa*. Historically, the hemp plant has had a wide range of uses, including making fiber, clothing, rope, and canvas. Hemp has been cultivated for thousands of years all over the world, including in the United States. Marijuana, hashish, and hash oil are all derived from hemp. All three forms are usually smoked and inhaled, although they're also sometimes eaten.

- What all of these forms of cannabis have in common is that they contain chemicals called cannabinoids. Many cannabinoids are psychoactive, so when they enter the bloodstream and get to the brain, they can produce psychological and behavioral effects.

- In 1964, scientists identified one particular cannabinoid that seems to be responsible for the major effects associated with marijuana use: delta-9-tetrahydrocannabinol (THC). It's the THC in hemp that produces many of the psychoactive effects associated with marijuana.

- How do cannabinoids like THC affect the brain? For a long time, we didn't know, but that changed in 1988, when William Devane, Allyn Howlett, and their colleagues at the St. Louis University medical school found evidence for cannabinoid receptors in the brain.

- Neurotransmitters bind to specific molecules called receptors in the brain, and most psychoactive drugs produce their effects by mimicking neurotransmitters and binding to natural brain receptors. Cannabinoids like THC are no exception to that rule. And the receptors that they bind to were even named after them; that's why they're called cannabinoid receptors.

- There are two major types of cannabinoid receptors in the body: the CB1 receptors and the CB2 receptors. The CB2 receptors play an important role in the immune system and are not thought to be involved in the psychological effects produced by marijuana. The CB1 receptors in the brain underlie those effects, so those are the receptors we'll focus on.

- Presumably, the brain doesn't have receptors that were specifically designed to respond to marijuana. Rather, scientists assumed that there must be some natural brain chemicals that bind to cannabinoid receptors. So, after discovering the receptors, scientists went looking for the chemicals, and in 1992, they found one, a natural brain chemical called anandamide. Subsequent studies have found a few others.

- These natural chemicals that are produced in the brain are sometimes called endogenous cannabinoids, or endocannabinoids. These are different from exogenous cannabinoids, which come from outside the body. Anandamide is an endocannabinoid because it is made within the body, while THC is an exogenous cannabinoid because it comes from outside—specifically from cannabis.

- When scientists investigated the properties of endogenous cannabinoids more deeply, they discovered that endocannabinoids are quite different than most other neurotransmitters in the brain. Most neurotransmitters are stored in neurons and then are released when the neuron fires, but endocannabinoids appear to be made only when they're needed rather than being stored.

- More importantly, cannabinoids seem to work largely as retrograde messengers. Recall that when neurons communicate, usually one of them fires and releases a bunch of neurotransmitter molecules into the synapse, or the small gap, between the cells. The neurotransmitter molecules then move across the synapse and bind to receptors on another neuron, perhaps causing that neuron to fire, too. The cell that fires and releases the neurotransmitter is called the presynaptic cell, and the cell that the neurotransmitter binds to is called the postsynaptic cell.

- Normally, brain chemicals move from the presynaptic cell and bind to receptors on the postsynaptic cell. But cannabinoid receptors are not usually found on the postsynaptic cell; instead, they're usually on the presynaptic cells. That led scientists to hypothesize that cannabinoids are typically used to send messages back from the postsynaptic cell to the presynaptic cell. That's what it means to be a retrograde messenger.

- Subsequent evidence has confirmed that hypothesis. In particular, endocannabinoids like anandamide are typically released by the postsynaptic cell and then move back to the presynaptic cell, where they bind to the CB1 receptors.

- Most scientists believe that retrograde messaging is used to regulate neural communication. Specifically, retrograde messaging can turn off the presynaptic cell once it has released enough neurotransmitter molecules and therefore prevent it from releasing too much. This mechanism has been found in both excitatory and inhibitory synapses, suggesting that cannabinoids can prevent too much excitation as well as too much inhibition.

- Furthermore, some recent evidence suggests that the regulatory functions of cannabinoids may be important in helping us forget things we need to forget. For example, suppose you park in the same structure that you parked in yesterday. Sometimes your memory of yesterday's parking spot can interfere with your ability to remember where you parked today. That's called proactive interference, and there's evidence that endocannabinoids can reduce this kind of interference. Likewise, cannabinoids are critical in unlearning fear, a phenomenon called fear extinction.

- These findings have led scientists in some interesting directions, such as using exogenous cannabinoids, including medical marijuana, to treat post-traumatic stress disorder (PTSD). These findings may also explain why marijuana users often report memory problems.

The Effects and Uses of Marijuana

- Cannabinoid receptors have been found all over the brain. They're found in areas involved in motor control and in areas that process fear and anxiety. They're also found in the midbrain dopamine system and the reward circuit. The fact that cannabinoid receptors are found in so many areas suggests that cannabinoids like THC might have a broad range of effects—and, in fact, they do.

- Marijuana users report a variety of effects that can differ substantially depending on the person and the situation. Many users report a feeling of euphoria and exhilaration as well as lowered inhibitions. Users also often report feeling relaxed and calm, and many experience enhanced visual and auditory perception. Some people also report a sense that time is slowing down substantially.

- At higher doses, marijuana can produce less-pleasant symptoms, such as disorganized thoughts and feelings of paranoia and anxiety. Higher doses are also associated with impaired judgment and agitation. However, there are no reported cases of death as a result of marijuana overdose, so in that sense, the margin of safety for marijuana seems to be much larger than the margin of safety for other drugs of abuse, such as heroin or cocaine.

- But besides these psychological effects, cannabinoids have other effects that have played an important role in their medicinal use. In particular, they can be quite effective in reducing nausea and vomiting and in increasing appetite, which are desirable in a number of circumstances, including treating many chronic illnesses, such as cancer and AIDS.

- In addition, cannabinoids have been shown to help relieve pain, particularly when traditional painkillers are insufficient. And there's even evidence from animal studies that cannabinoids may inhibit the development of certain types of tumors.

- There are some legitimate medical uses of cannabinoids. Indeed, there are now cannabinoid-based pills that are approved for use in the treatment of both chemotherapy-induced nausea and AIDS. In many states, medical marijuana has been legalized and is being used to treat patients. In fact, in 2012, Colorado and Washington State even legalized the recreational use of marijuana.

- On the other hand, there are often alternative drugs that can treat the same symptoms without the psychoactive effects of cannabinoids. For example, synthetic derivatives of the hormone progesterone

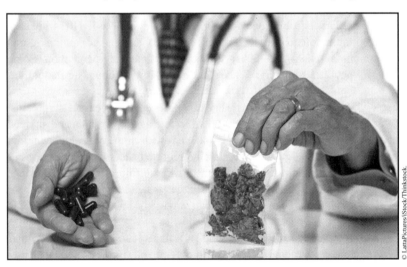

© LattaPictures/iStock/Thinkstock.

Cannabinoids can be effective in reducing nausea and vomiting and in increasing appetite, which is desirable in treating many chronic illnesses.

also increase appetite, and some studies suggest that they actually do so more effectively than cannabinoids. In short, the debate over medical marijuana isn't over yet.

Marijuana Addiction and Abuse

- Marijuana is the most widely used illegal drug in the world. More than 17 million Americans use marijuana in a typical month, and there are more than 3 million daily users. Marijuana use typically starts during adolescence. Among high school seniors, about one-third have used marijuana during the past year and about one-fifth are current users. In fact, about one in eight eighth graders have reported trying marijuana in the past year. But does trying marijuana lead to chronic use?

- A 1994 survey conducted by the National Institute on Drug Abuse found that about nine percent of people who tried marijuana at least once eventually became addicted. This number is significant, but it's also lower than the addiction rates for other drugs that were evaluated in the survey. Marijuana is indeed somewhat addictive, but it's not as addictive as most other drugs of abuse. Work with animals also suggests that marijuana, and exogenous cannabinoids in general, are moderately addictive.

- The mechanisms of addiction are also at work with marijuana. Specifically, like other drugs of abuse, marijuana has been shown to lead to enhanced activity in the reward circuit and to stimulate the firing of dopamine neurons in the ventral tegmental area. Furthermore, injections of the endogenous cannabinoid anandamide have been shown to produce pleasurable reactions in animals.

- In addition, there is some evidence that chronic marijuana users develop a physical dependence on the drug. Specifically, when they stop using marijuana, they often exhibit withdrawal symptoms, including craving, irritability, anxiety, depression, and reduced appetite.

- However, the evidence for the development of tolerance is mixed. On one hand, we have evidence for tolerance at a physiological level, in terms of a reduction in the number of receptors. But on the other hand, the evidence for behavioral tolerance is much weaker.

Consequences of Marijuana Use

- There are some negative consequences associated with chronic marijuana use. For example, compared with nonsmoking peers, students who regularly smoke marijuana tend to get lower grades, and they're also more likely to drop out of high school. However, these studies are correlational in nature, and correlational studies do not support claims about causality. In other words, just because marijuana use is correlated with poor academic performance, that doesn't mean that marijuana use caused the poor grades.

- There's also good evidence for a correlation between marijuana use and what is sometimes called an amotivational syndrome. That is, chronic marijuana users are often more apathetic or aimless than nonusers, and they may lack motivation and exhibit decreased productivity in general. Again, we have a correlation between marijuana use and these behaviors, but we have not established causation.

- There's also controversy about whether marijuana might be a gateway to harder drugs. The gateway theory claims that marijuana use primes the pump and puts one at risk for the use of more dangerous drugs, such as cocaine and heroin, later in life. While early marijuana use is indeed associated with later use of harder drugs, once again that correlation doesn't necessarily imply causation.

- Another potential negative consequence of marijuana use is your health. The health effects of marijuana don't seem to be as bad as the health effects of alcohol and cigarettes. Long-term use does seem to be associated with bronchitis, and marijuana smoke actually contains higher concentrations of some carcinogens than cigarette smoke does, but the link between chronic marijuana use and lung cancer has not yet been conclusively demonstrated.

Treatment for Marijuana Addiction

- Most current treatments for marijuana addiction use behavioral therapy. In particular, many techniques combine cognitive behavioral therapy with motivational incentives. Cognitive behavioral therapy trains patients to recognize and avoid the triggers associated with cravings and teaches them strategies to cope with those cravings without using. Many therapies also include a motivational component, in which patients are rewarded, sometimes even with money, for abstinence.

- There is evidence that these techniques can help. For example, in one study, 37 percent of people who received cognitive behavioral therapy along with motivational incentives remained abstinent after one year. In comparison, only 17 percent of people who received motivational incentives alone managed to remain abstinent. Likewise, only 23 percent of people who received cognitive behavioral therapy alone remained abstinent. Like most other addictions, we don't yet have particularly effective approaches to treating marijuana addiction.

Suggested Reading

Compton, Grant, Colliver, Glantz, and Stinson, "Prevalence of Marijuana Use Disorders in the United States."

Earleywine, *Understanding Marijuana.*

Iverson, *The Science of Marijuana.*

Questions to Consider

1. What are some of the functions of endogenous cannabinoids?

2. What are some of the potential medical uses of cannabinoids?

3. Do you think that marijuana should be legalized for medical use, or even recreational use? Why, or why not?

Stimulants—From Cocaine to Ritalin
Lecture 9

In this lecture, you will learn about stimulant drugs, which are sometimes colloquially referred to as "uppers" because they produce a feeling of excitement and euphoria, increase alertness and focus, and decrease fatigue and appetite. Cocaine, amphetamine, and methamphetamine all belong to this class of drugs and are often considered among the most dangerous drugs of abuse available. In this lecture, you will learn background information on psychostimulants. You also will learn about what kinds of effects these drugs have, especially on the brain, and about addiction, abuse, and treatment.

The History of Psychostimulants

- Like many other drugs of abuse, cocaine comes from a plant. Specifically, it comes from the coca plant, which is prevalent in the countries of Colombia, Peru, and Bolivia in South America. And just like caffeine and nicotine, cocaine is thought to act as a natural insecticide for the coca plant, to prevent bugs from eating it.

- The people living in the regions where the coca plant grows have known that the plant has stimulating effects for thousands of years. And many people in these regions regularly chew coca leaves for these effects. Cocaine ingested this way reaches the brain slowly over a long period of time, so the effects are much milder than snorting cocaine powder or smoking cocaine in the form of crack.

- But in the mid-1800s, German chemists isolated cocaine in its pure form, and its use—and abuse—really took off. By the beginning of the 20th century, people began to realize that cocaine was both addictive and potentially very harmful. In 1914, the U.S. Congress passed legislation imposing restrictions on its use and sale.

- Cocaine comes in a number of different forms. The most familiar is probably cocaine powder, which is a water-soluble salt called cocaine hydrochloride. This form of cocaine is often snorted. In the 1970s, some users began treating cocaine powder with chemicals and freeing the cocaine base from the hydrochloride salt in a process called freebasing. The resulting freebase cocaine melts at a lower temperature, which means it can be smoked. And that gets the cocaine to the brain faster and produces a more intense high. However, freebasing involves the use of highly flammable solvents, so it can be dangerous.

- Around 1980, a dried, hardened version of cocaine called crack cocaine appeared. Crack cocaine can also be smoked, leading to a similar very intense high and strong potential for abuse, but its production doesn't involve the use of flammable solvents, so there's less risk of an accident.

- The histories of amphetamine and methamphetamine are similar to the history of cocaine. Like cocaine, amphetamines are also derived from a plant—in this case, the *Ephedra sinica* plant, which grows mainly in Mongolia, Russia, and Northeast China. And like the coca plant, the ephedra plant has been used for thousands of years by people who recognized its effects. Specifically, it has played an important part in traditional Chinese medicine as a treatment for colds and asthma.

- In the late 1800s, chemists synthesized amphetamine from the ephedra plant. About 30 years later, they synthesized methamphetamine. Both are potent and addictive psychostimulants, but methamphetamine tends to have stronger effects because of a slight change in chemical structure.

- For a long time, amphetamine was used to treat nasal congestion and head colds, under the trade name Benzedrine. In 1937, the American Medical Association sanctioned the use of amphetamine for the treatment of mild depression and sleep disorders. Amphetamine was even a common diet pill in the 1940s.

- Stimulants also played an important role during World War II, when many soldiers took them in order to stay awake and alert. After World War II, the use of amphetamines in the general population really grew. For example, in 1970, over 10 billion amphetamine tablets were legally made in the United States.

- But probably the most widespread legal use of amphetamines in the United States has been in the treatment of attention deficit disorder (ADD) and attention deficit/hyperactivity disorder (ADHD). The two most-common drugs used in the treatment of these disorders are Adderall and Ritalin, both of which are psychostimulants. By 2014, roughly 3 million children in the United States were taking one of these medications to treat ADD or ADHD.

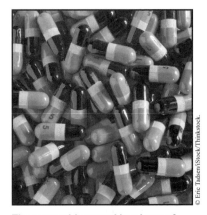

- Because low doses of psychostimulants improve focus, these drugs have been found to help sufferers stay on task and get their work done. It's also important to note that when used as directed, these medications are quite safe. Studies have found that when used as directed, the potential for addiction and abuse is quite low. Unfortunately, these drugs aren't always used as directed.

The most widespread legal use of amphetamines in the United States is in the treatment of ADD and ADHD.

- Methamphetamine is perhaps the most dangerous of all the psychostimulant drugs. The methamphetamine molecule is just an amphetamine molecule with an additional methyl group, consisting of a carbon atom and three hydrogen atoms. That change may seem minor, but the additional methyl group makes methamphetamine much more likely to be abused.

- One reason is that the extra methyl group makes it easier for methamphetamine to get to the brain compared with standard amphetamine. More of it can reach the brain, and it can produce a larger effect that lasts much longer. Another reason methamphetamine has become popular among recreational drug users is that it's relatively easy to make using widely available chemicals, such as the pseudoephedrine found in decongestants.

- In an attempt to slow down the illegal manufacture of methamphetamine, Congress passed an act called the Combat Methamphetamine Epidemic Act of 2005, which required that cold medicines containing pseudoephedrine be kept behind the counter. Anyone buying those medicines had to present a photo identification, and the amount they could buy was limited and tracked.

- The most potent form of methamphetamine is crystal meth, which users often call glass or ice. Like crack cocaine, it's usually smoked and produces a very intense high. But that high typically lasts much longer than the high from other stimulants. Users therefore see it as a very cost-effective drug, because a small dose can go a long way.

The Effects of Psychostimulants

- As their name suggests, stimulant drugs stimulate the nervous system. And that stimulation has some positive effects: It reduces fatigue, increases alertness, and produces feelings of excitement and euphoria. Unfortunately, the negative consequences of these drugs can be disastrous.

- For example, in addition to its stimulating psychological effects, cocaine also constricts blood vessels, meaning that less blood can reach critical organs, such as the brain and heart, resulting in strokes and associated brain damage and heart attacks.

- In addition to posing a serious health risk, high doses of psychostimulants also sometimes lead to stereotypic behavior, which is repetitive movements such as body rocking, crossing and uncrossing legs, or marching in place.

- Chronic stimulant use can also sometimes lead to psychosis, including vivid hallucinations and delusions. The user might develop extreme paranoia and experience delusions of being followed or persecuted. Users also commonly claim that they feel imaginary insects burrowing under their skin, so they compulsively pick and scratch at themselves. As a result, they often have scars and lesions all over their body.

- How do psychostimulants affect the brain? All psychostimulants directly increase dopamine levels in the brain. Dopamine plays a central role in craving and addiction. Nicotine, alcohol, and marijuana all lead to the release of dopamine, but these other drugs do so indirectly. Psychostimulants increase dopamine levels directly, which might be a reason why they're among the most abused drugs in the world.

- The way they work is also somewhat different from the other drugs discussed so far. Recall how neurons communicate using neurotransmitter molecules: When the presynaptic neuron fires, it releases neurotransmitter molecules into the synapse, and those molecules then bind to receptors on the postsynaptic neuron, like a key fitting into a lock. But what happens to those neurotransmitter molecules after they've done their work?

- One thing that happens is that the neurotransmitter molecules can be sucked back into the presynaptic cell by molecules called transporters. This way, the neurotransmitter molecules can be used again when the neuron fires again. This process is called reuptake, because the neurotransmitter molecules are taken back up into the presynaptic neuron.

- Most of the drugs of abuse discussed so far mimic the actions of neurotransmitters and bind to receptors. They may activate those receptors if they're agonists, or they may block those receptors if they're antagonists. But psychostimulants work differently. Rather than binding to receptors, psychostimulants typically affect the cell's transporters.

- Rather than sucking the dopamine out of the synapse, the transporter molecules are now spraying dopamine back into the synapse, resulting in much higher levels of dopamine than normal. In fact, some studies have found that cocaine can lead to double the normal amount of dopamine in the synapse, and methamphetamine can produce a tenfold increase in dopamine levels.

Addiction to Psychostimulants

- Cocaine and methamphetamine are among the most addictive drugs in the world, especially when they're smoked or injected. All animal species that have been tested will self-administer these drugs intravenously, and they'll do so compulsively.

- Human addicts often exhibit bingeing behavior with psychostimulants, especially crack cocaine and crystal meth. After taking an initial dose, they experience an intense high and euphoria, but as soon as that high starts to wear off, they administer another dose to try to keep the high going and avoid coming down. They might repeat this cycle for days without eating or sleeping, until they finally run out of the drug or crash from exhaustion.

- Like most other drugs of abuse that have been discussed, repeated use of psychostimulants leads to changes in the brain that make it harder and harder to resist the drug. Repeated use of psychostimulants leads to tolerance; it takes more of the drug to produce the same effect.

- Psychostimulants are thought to be addictive for the same reasons as other drugs. The drugs produce a large release of dopamine and overstimulate the brain's reward circuit. That dopamine produces craving and signals a reward prediction error, which backs up to cues associated with the drug taking. With repeated use, many environmental cues become extremely strong triggers that lead to irresistible cravings for the drug, and an addiction is born.

Treatments for Psychostimulant Addictions

- Currently, behavioral approaches are the treatment of choice for psychostimulant addictions. One approach is called contingency management, or motivational incentives. In these kinds of programs, addicts receive points or chips for each drug-free urine test. And they can then redeem these points for rewards like movie tickets or dinner at a restaurant. This kind of approach has been found to be effective in achieving initial abstinence and in sticking with treatment.

- Another approach called cognitive behavioral therapy is helpful in preventing relapse. Essentially, addicts are taught to recognize risky situations that could trigger relapse and avoid those situations as much as possible. They're also taught coping skills to help them deal with cravings when they arise.

- Many addicts also find community-based recovery groups like Cocaine Anonymous to be helpful as a support system when trying to remain abstinent, or to get back on the wagon after relapse. Other addicts benefit from residential programs, where they live in a community of recovering addicts for six months or more.

- Unfortunately, relapse rates are quite high. For example, around 90 percent of methamphetamine addicts have been estimated to return to using after treatment. It's therefore particularly important for stimulant addicts to keep trying and to view relapses as learning opportunities in their journey to achieve complete abstinence eventually.

- There are currently no pharmacological treatments that are approved to treat psychostimulant addiction; however, scientists have been working on vaccines that could potentially help addicts avoid relapse. The idea is to train the body's own immune system to recognize and attack cocaine and methamphetamine before they reach the brain. So, even if an addict who is in recovery falls off the wagon, much less of the drug would reach the brain, and they would not experience the normal high.

Suggested Reading

Center for Substance Abuse Treatment, "How Stimulants Affect the Brain and Behavior."

Markel, *An Anatomy of Addiction*.

Moore, *The Amphetamine Debate*.

Sheff, *Beautiful Boy*.

Questions to Consider

1. How were cocaine and amphetamines used before they were regulated?

2. How does cocaine influence neural function?

3. Do you think that it's okay to use stimulants in the treatment of ADHD?

The Science of Poppies, Pleasure, and Pain
Lecture 10

This lecture tells the story of the poppy plant. In addition to producing beautiful flowers and edible seeds, the poppy plant is also the source of opium and the many drugs derived from opium. Among these drugs are medicines that have revolutionized the treatment of pain, such as codeine and morphine, as well as heroin, which is often considered to be the most harmful drug of abuse today. Although opioid drugs are very addictive, they are nevertheless very effective painkillers and are still widely used in medicine.

Opium

- Opium is actually a kind of dried latex, which is a milky fluid that is secreted by some plants when they're damaged, as a defense mechanism against insects trying to eat them. Opium is the latex secreted from the seedpod of an opium poppy. Raw opium contains about 10 percent morphine and about 2 percent codeine. These are the opiate drugs, which just means that they're natural products of the opium poppy. A number of other drugs, including heroin, are not contained in opium itself but are made from natural opiates or have very similar effects. These are sometimes called opioids.

- The opiate drug morphine is among the most effective painkillers available today. Codeine has similar effects but is weaker than morphine. It's often used to treat minor pain and as a cough suppressant. Of course, opium and drugs derived from opium are also often used recreationally, because they can produce a dreamlike, euphoric state.

- People have known about those effects for a very long time. In fact, there's evidence that the Sumerians knew about the psychoactive properties of the opium poppy plant as early as 3400 B.C. The

Ancient Egyptians used opium medicinally. In the 1700s and 1800s, a mixture of alcohol and opium called laudanum became very popular and was widely used as a pain reliever, as a sleep aid, and to treat a variety of ailments. In the mid-1800s opium trade became a big business and even led to two wars, known as the opium wars, between the British and the Chinese.

- In 1804, a German pharmacist isolated a pure alkaloid from opium and gave it the name morphine, after Morpheus, the Greek god of dreams. Morphine was more potent than opium or laudanum, and it became an invaluable tool to doctors in the treatment of pain. Morphine was administered to injured soldiers during the American Civil War.

- In 1898, Bayer pharmaceutical company began selling a synthesized opioid that was one-and-a-half to two times more powerful than morphine, and it was marketed as a nonaddictive morphine

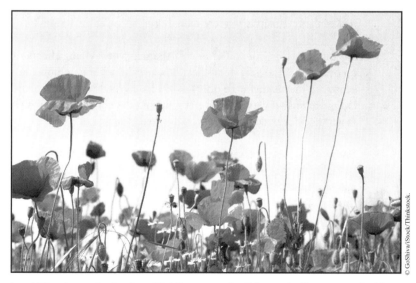

In addition to producing beautiful flowers and edible seeds, the poppy plant is also the source of opium and the many drugs derived from opium.

substitute and cough suppressant—heroin. Bayer sold heroin for more than 10 years before its harmful effects were recognized and it was removed from the market. Heroin is now recognized to be among the most addictive drugs in the world.

• Today, a wide variety of opioid medications are available as prescription painkillers. Vicodin, Percocet, Fentanyl, Methadone, and OxyContin are all examples of opioids that are used to relieve chronic pain, and they're prescribed a lot. Although these medications are extremely effective, they're also potentially addictive, and a large number of people who begin using them for pain relief eventually get hooked.

The Effects of Opioids on Behavior and the Brain

• Opioids are narcotic analgesics, which reduce pain without eliminating sensation. They're distinguished from anesthetics, which reduce all sensation and often produce unconsciousness. Opioids also produce a dreamlike, euphoric state, which is what makes them attractive to recreational drug users, at least initially.

• At low doses, pain relief is one of the main behavioral effects of opioids. And the fact that they block pain without eliminating sensation makes them the drugs of choice in the treatment of pain. Opioids are also very effective at reducing the cough reflex, which is why they're widely used as cough suppressants.

• Some of the less-pleasant effects include nausea and constipation. In fact, constipation is one of the biggest problems in the long-term use of opioids to treat chronic pain. On the other hand, this means that opioids can also be used as a treatment for diarrhea.

• At higher doses, opioids produce a rush of euphoria. But the nauseating effects can become more severe, and some people also experience anxiety and restlessness. The most dangerous effect is a significant suppression of breathing. In fact, in an opioid overdose, breathing can be suppressed enough to lead to death.

- What's going on in the brain and the body that makes opioids so powerful? Like almost all the other drugs of abuse that have been discussed, opioids work by binding to receptors. There are a number of different types of opioid receptors, but it's the mu-opioid receptors that seem to be the most important in producing the behavioral effects just discussed.

- Mu-opioid receptors have a high affinity for morphine and related drugs, meaning that these drugs bind very strongly and take longer to dissociate. As a result, the drugs can be quite potent. Mu-opioid receptors are found in the places that you might expect based on the behavioral effects that opioids produce, including in the brain and gastrointestinal tract.

- Like in the case of marijuana, scientists found the opioid receptors before they found any of the endogenous brain chemicals that bind to those receptors. In fact, they found three major types of endogenous opioids: the dynorphins, the enkephalins, and the endorphins. You may recall that chronic drug use leads to the release of dynorphins in order to inhibit ventral tegmental area (VTA) neurons and prevent them from exciting the nucleus accumbens, and that contributes to tolerance to the pleasurable effects of drugs.

- The enkephalins and the endorphins are both natural painkillers, but they're active in different parts of the body. When you're injured or in pain, your body releases these chemicals, and they help block the pain. Endorphins are morphine-like substances, but they originate in the brain itself. In addition to being released during pain, endorphins are also released during stress and strenuous exercise and when you're eating spicy food. When they're released, they activate the mu-opioid

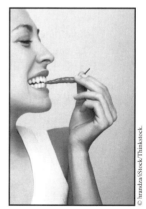

© brandzai/iStock/Thinkstock.

Endorphins are released when you experience pain and eat spicy food.

receptors, just like morphine does. They therefore relieve pain and produce a pleasurable high, basically the same symptoms as morphine.

Opioid Abuse

- About 45 people in the United States die every day from overdosing on a prescription painkiller—that's more than the number of overdose deaths from heroin and cocaine combined. What's going on in the brain that might lead to addiction to opioids?

- Similar to other drugs, opioids overstimulate the brain's reward circuit and trigger a large release of dopamine. The brain interprets that dopamine as a reward prediction error, or an indication that taking the drug was better than expected. That reward prediction error in turn backs up to environmental cues that are associated with drug taking, so when the user encounters those cues in the future, he or she experiences a very strong craving to use the drug.

- How do we know that the same mechanisms underlie addiction to opium? The VTA is the part of the reward circuit that contains dopamine neurons. Scientists have found that injecting opioids into the VTA leads to increased dopamine cell firing and a release of dopamine into the nucleus accumbens. Opioids do this by inhibiting the neurons that inhibit the VTA. In other words, opioids disinhibit the VTA, which makes those neurons fire more and leads to dopamine release. This same kind of disinhibition mechanism is at work with alcohol.

- Furthermore, scientists have found that applying a dopamine receptor antagonist, which blocks the effect of dopamine, also blocks the reinforcing effects of opioids. Animals taking these dopamine receptor antagonists don't develop addictions to opioids like other animals do, which demonstrates that dopamine is once again playing a central role.

Treatment for Opioid Abuse and Addiction

- There are some very effective treatments for opioid overdose. Specifically, a number of opioid receptor antagonist drugs have been developed that have a high affinity for opioid receptors but that don't actually activate them. These drugs can therefore block opioids from binding to the receptors.

- If a drug user overdoses on opioids, is barely breathing, and is close to death, if someone administers one of these opioid antagonist drugs, such as naloxone, the drug user will recover almost immediately, because the opioid will be blocked from binding to the opioid receptors.

- But that's just treating the overdose. What about the addiction? Detoxification is the first step to helping opioid addicts quit the habit. But detoxification can be a real challenge for opioid addicts because users experience very unpleasant withdrawal symptoms when they stop taking the drug. The symptoms are the mirror opposite of the effects produced by the drug itself: Instead of euphoria, withdrawal is characterized by depression; instead of pain relief, withdrawal leads to aches and pains; and instead of constipation, withdrawal produces diarrhea.

- A common approach to treating opioid addiction is to administer a slower, longer-acting opioid, such as methadone, instead. In fact, methadone maintenance is the single most-common treatment for heroin addiction, and it has had significant success. For example, one study found that 80 percent of people who stick with a methadone maintenance program for a full year end up staying abstinent for one to three years afterward. In contrast, only 12 percent of people who drop out of methadone maintenance remain abstinent for that long.

- Other opioids are also regularly used in the treatment of heroin addiction. In fact, heroin itself is used in the treatment of heroin addiction in a number of countries. The idea is to give users a lower, but stable, prescription dose of heroin without all the risks associated with obtaining and using heroin on the street. Not surprisingly, heroin addicts are more likely to stick with a heroin maintenance program compared with a methadone maintenance program, and perhaps as a result, they're less likely to use illegal drugs.

- Using opioid drugs like methadone to treat heroin addicts is controversial. After all, you're simply substituting one addiction for another. Another problem is that the addicts have to go to a clinic every day or two in order to receive their treatment, and the people living near the clinics don't particularly like the large traffic of heroin addicts who are coming to the neighborhood every day.

- Another common approach to treating opioid addiction is to try to remove any reward associated with relapse. Sometimes, addicts who have managed to quit will take an opioid antagonist like naltrexone, which blocks the rewarding effects of any opioids they take. The idea is that if they ever get a strong craving and end up using an opioid drug, they won't experience their normal high because of the antagonist that's in their system. This can work well for somebody who's very motivated to quit. The problem is that people who experience very strong cravings may just stop taking the antagonist drug so that they can get the high again.

- In most cases, these kinds of pharmacological treatments are most effective if they're combined with some sort of behavioral treatment. It's very helpful for opioid addicts to get some kind of cognitive behavioral therapy in which they're trained to recognize and avoid the triggers that they associate with drug use. They're also taught coping skills to help them deal with the cravings when they do arise. Furthermore, 12-step programs like Narcotics Anonymous can be helpful for a number of people.

- However, breaking a drug addiction is tough, and breaking an addiction to an opioid is among the toughest challenges anyone will ever face. But as with all addictions, it's important to keep in mind that one relapse does not mean failure. It simply represents an opportunity for the addict to learn from the experience and hopefully be successful the next time.

Suggested Reading

Akil, Watson, Young, Lewis, Khachaturian, and Walker, "Endogenous Opioids."

Christie, "Cellular Neuroadaptations to Chronic Opioids."

Fernandez and Libby, *Heroin*.

Martin, *Opium Fiend*.

Questions to Consider

1. What are some of the major opioid drugs?

2. What are some of the major functions of endogenous opioids?

3. Do you think that addictive drugs should be used in the treatment of other addictions?

The Gambler's Brain
Lecture 11

I n this lecture, you will be introduced to the scientific evidence of similarities in the behavior, the brain, and even the genes of compulsive gamblers and drug addicts. As you will learn, scientists are starting to view problem gambling as another type of addiction—but, in this case, it's an addiction to a behavior rather than a drug. This implies that we can no longer think of an addiction simply as a dependence on a particular chemical. Instead, any activity that hyperstimulates the brain's reward circuit could potentially be addictive.

Gambling versus Drugs of Abuse: Behavioral Symptoms

- Gambling is sometimes defined as putting something of value— usually money—at risk in the hopes of getting something of greater value. According to American Gaming Association statistics, commercial casinos in America earn more than 35 billion dollars every year. Likewise, revenue in gaming facilities on Indian reservations exceeds 25 billion dollars per year. And those numbers don't even include Internet gambling, which is the fastest growing part of the industry.

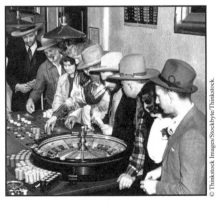

Any activity that hyperstimulates the brain's reward circuit—like gambling, for example—could potentially be addictive.

- About 85 percent of U.S. adults have gambled occasionally in their lives, and the vast majority don't experience any significant problems. However, an estimated 4 to 6 million people in the

United States experience problems as a result of their gambling, and about 2 million meet the criteria for pathological gambling or gambling disorder.

- For a long time, psychiatrists considered pathological gambling to be primarily a problem with impulse control, rather than an addiction. Now, gambling disorder is classified as a behavioral addiction, based on studies demonstrating that pathological gambling and drug addiction share a number of similarities, ranging from similar behavioral symptoms to similar neural substrates—and even similar genetic profiles.

- Both drug addiction and pathological gambling are characterized by persistence in the behavior despite negative consequences and an inability to stop. The Diagnostic and Statistical Manual of Mental Disorders, the standard classification of mental disorders, provides lists of symptoms that mental health professionals have identified as robust behavioral features that should be considered when diagnosing a disorder. The lists of behavioral symptoms associated with drug addiction and with gambling disorder are remarkably similar.

- For example, one of the behavioral symptoms associated with drug addiction is "recurrent substance use resulting in a failure to fulfill major role obligations at work, school, or home." Similarly, one of the behavioral criteria for diagnosing gambling disorder is whether the person "has jeopardized or lost a significant relationship, job, or educational or career opportunity because of gambling."

- Another behavioral symptom of drug addiction is "persistent desire or unsuccessful efforts to cut down or control substance use." Again, similarly, another one of the symptoms associated with gambling disorder is "has made repeated unsuccessful efforts to control, cut back, or stop gambling."

- Evidence suggests that compulsive gamblers experience symptoms of tolerance and withdrawal, too. For example, Dr. Mark Griffiths measured the heart rate of 30 young men at the University of

Plymouth while they played slot machines. Half the men were regular gamblers, and the other half were not. Griffiths found that everyone's heart rate increased when they started playing the game, suggesting that they were experiencing a rush of excitement. But after they stopped playing, the heart rate of the gamblers quickly dropped back down, while the heart rate of the non-gamblers remained high.

- Griffiths suggested that the rush associated with gambling wore off more quickly in experienced gamblers, reflecting tolerance to the rewarding aspects of the behavior. Consistent with this interpretation, chronic gamblers often need to gamble larger amounts of money to feel the same rush of excitement, much like drug addicts need more of the drug to feel high.

- Many chronic gamblers also appear to experience withdrawal when they stop gambling. Richard Rosenthal at the UCLA Gambling Studies Program, along with Henry Lesieur, asked 222 pathological gamblers about symptoms they experienced when they tried to slow down or stop gambling. Ninety-one percent said that they experienced cravings, and 87 percent felt restless and irritable. Two-thirds even reported physical symptoms, such as headaches, insomnia, sweating, and shaking.

Gambling versus Drugs of Abuse: Neural Mechanisms
- Chronic drug use tends to lead to a numbing of response in the brain's pleasure center, the nucleus accumbens. In addition, drugs of abuse trigger a large release of dopamine into the reward circuit, which over time leads to strong associations between drug-related cues and drug taking, resulting in strong craving. Furthermore, chronic drug use is associated with reduced self-control as a result of weakened inhibitory input from the prefrontal cortex.

- Jan Reuter, Christian Büchel, and their colleagues at the University of Hamburg used functional magnetic resonance imaging (fMRI) to estimate neural activity in pathological gamblers and in control subjects while they performed a very simple gambling task.

They found that the reward response is numbed in pathological gamblers, just like it is in drug addicts. In addition, they found that the most severe gamblers also had the most numbed reward response.

- So, chronic gambling is indeed associated with reduced activation of the nucleus accumbens and a numbed reward response, just like drug addiction. Furthermore, as the reward response becomes more and more numb, the gambling problem becomes worse, perhaps because the gamblers need to gamble more to feel the same level of excitement and reward.

- Another brain change that occurs with drug addiction is the large dopamine burst in response to drug-related cues and an associated craving whenever those cues were encountered. Anna Goudriaan and colleagues at the University of Amsterdam investigated evidence for a similar brain change in chronic gambling in an experiment in 2010. They used fMRI to estimate neural activity while pathological gamblers and control subjects viewed different kinds of pictures, some related to gambling and others not.

- They found neural evidence that the gamblers were sensitized to gambling-related cues. Furthermore, that increased sensitivity was associated with craving. This is exactly what is assumed to be happening in drug addiction, too.

- One thing this study doesn't tell us is whether dopamine is involved. Functional MRI really only tells you about neural activity, so it's impossible to know whether dopamine was actually being released when the gambling-related cues were presented. But there is some evidence for that hypothesis. In fact, patients with Parkinson's disease who are taking dopamine agonists are roughly three times more likely to become pathological gamblers than people who aren't taking these drugs. So, it seems like dopamine plays a role in the development of gambling addiction.

- A third brain change that is associated with drug addiction is reduced inhibitory control from prefrontal cortex. Evidence suggests that pathological gamblers also exhibit reduced prefrontal activity and an associated deficit in the ability to inhibit inappropriate behavior. In fact, gamblers behave a lot like patients with damage to their prefrontal cortex.

- Marc Potenza and colleagues at the Yale University School of Medicine have found direct evidence for reduced prefrontal activity in pathological gamblers. They used fMRI to estimate neural activity while pathological gamblers and control subjects exerted self-control. They found that activation of the prefrontal cortex was significantly reduced in the pathological gamblers compared with non-gamblers, and they interpreted this result as evidence for an impairment in prefrontal inhibitory control—which is the same kind of impairment that is present in drug addicts.

Gambling versus Drugs of Abuse: Genetics
- Drug addiction, and the traits associated with drug addiction, are all significantly heritable. The same is true of pathological gambling. The heritability of a trait is typically estimated by comparing the similarity of that trait in identical twins with the similarity in fraternal twins. Dr. Seth Eisen at the Washington University School of Medicine and his colleagues used this approach to estimate the heritability of pathological gambling.

- They found that identical twins were much more likely to be similar in terms of pathological gambling than were fraternal twins. In fact, they estimated pathological gambling to be 62 percent heritable, meaning that more than half of the variation in gambling diagnosis was based on genetics rather than environment.

- So, both drug addiction and pathological gambling are heritable. In fact, it appears that some of the same genes are involved. Evidence for this comes from investigating the so-called comorbidity, or co-occurrence, of pathological gambling with drug addiction. Pathological gambling and drug addiction tend to co-occur in the same people surprisingly often, which suggests that some of the same genetic factors are at work. This comorbidity is particularly high for gambling and alcoholism.

- Dr. Wendy Slutske at the University of Missouri, along with a number of colleagues, analyzed the data from thousands of twins to assess the relationship between pathological gambling and alcoholism quantitatively, and they concluded that there must be at least one shared genetic factor that increases susceptibility for both pathological gambling and alcoholism.

- What might that genetic factor be? There's a lot more that scientists don't yet know about that question than they do know, but there are a few candidate genes that have been discovered. Perhaps the most promising is one of the dopamine receptor genes.

- Recall that genes code for specific proteins and that different versions of the same gene lead to different versions of those proteins. A variation in the gene that codes for one type of dopamine receptor has been found to be associated with pathological gambling as well as many types of drug addiction. This gene is typically called the DRD2 gene, which just means that it codes for the D2 type of dopamine receptor.

- Why would one form of this gene increase risk for addiction? The risky form is associated with what's sometimes called a reward deficiency syndrome. The idea is that people who have this genetic variant need more stimulation to experience the same level of reward and satisfaction as people who don't have it. People with this genetic variant might be particularly drawn to drugs because drugs are one of the only things that can stimulate their numbed reward circuit. These people are therefore more susceptible to addiction than other people.

- Consistent with this theory, people with this genetic variant are more likely to get addicted to cigarettes, alcohol, and other drugs of abuse. They're also more likely to become pathological gamblers. That is, the same gene that confers risk for alcoholism, nicotine dependence, and cocaine addiction also confers risk for pathological gambling.

Treatment for Gambling
- Some of the same approaches that are used in the treatment of drug addictions are also used in the treatment of pathological gambling, which may not be surprising given all the similarities they share. For example, many people find 12-step programs like Gamblers Anonymous to be helpful, because they provide social support and accountability from people who can understand and relate.

- Another approach is cognitive behavioral therapy. The basic idea behind this type of therapy is that our behavior is a result of our thoughts, so if we can identify the thoughts and motivations that give rise to gambling, then we can begin to control it. Once a gambler has developed an explicit strategy, he or she is much better equipped to cope with the urges to gamble when they arise.

- Somewhat surprisingly, certain medical treatments that have been used for drug and alcohol addiction have also proved helpful in treating gambling addiction. In particular, a number of studies have found that the opioid antagonist naltrexone, which is a treatment for alcohol, is also effective in reducing gambling behavior.

- Why would an opioid antagonist help reduce gambling and gambling urges? Opioids activate the nucleus accumbens and produce feelings of euphoria. Being an opioid antagonist, naltrexone competes with endogenous opioids and therefore blocks the high associated with gambling. And blocking that high makes gambling less appealing and therefore easier to resist.

Suggested Reading

Blum, Cull, Braverman, and Comings, "Reward Deficiency Syndrome."

el-Guebaly, Mudry, Zohar, Tavares, and Potenza, "Compulsive Features in Behavioural Addictions."

Grant and Potenza, eds., *Pathological Gambling.*

Potenza, "Neurobiology of Gambling Behaviors."

Schüll, *Addiction by Design.*

Questions to Consider

1. What are some of the major behavioral similarities between pathological gambling and drug addiction?

2. What are some of the major neural similarities between pathological gambling and drug addiction?

3. Do you think that gambling should be legal or illegal?

Junk Food, Porn, Video Games—Addictions?
Lecture 12

There are many behaviors that people persistently engage in despite significant negative consequences, and some of these behaviors may involve the consumption of a stimulus other than a drug. In this lecture, you will learn about three such stimuli: junk food, pornography, and video games. Specifically, you will learn about the psychology of these stimuli and the ways in which they are supernormal, meaning that they exaggerate features of normal stimuli that human beings were designed to find rewarding. In addition, you will learn about the neuroscience of these supernormal stimuli and whether their neural effects are similar to the effects of drugs of abuse.

Junk Food

- Obesity is a significant health problem in the United States. In fact, about two-thirds of Americans are overweight and about one-third are clinically obese. There are a number of reasons for the epidemic of obesity in the United States, but one of the most important reasons is the easy access to junk food.

- For almost all of human history, people had no choice but to eat fresh, unprocessed food that was relatively low in calories. There simply weren't any alternatives; high-calorie foods were very rare. Furthermore, most people had to walk long distances and perform quite a bit of manual labor just to survive. They therefore burned a lot of calories relatively quickly.

- In these kinds of environments, calories are a precious commodity, so it's important for us to be motivated to consume high-calorie foods whenever we can. And our brains are designed to do just that. Foods that are high in sugar, fat, or salt can taste very good and be very rewarding. In fact, motivating us to consume high-calorie foods is one of the things our reward circuit was designed for. And for most of our history, being motivated to eat high-calorie foods was a very good thing, because it inspired us to get as many precious calories as possible.

- The problem is that in Western society today, calories aren't nearly so precious. In fact, they're very easy to come by. High-calorie foods for our ancestors included foods like fruit and nuts. But today, we have high-fat junk foods and refined carbohydrates. These kinds of foods have far more calories than anything our ancestors would have eaten, so the motivational circuits in our brains find them extremely rewarding.

- Junk foods are supernormal stimuli—exaggerated versions of our ancestors' fruits and nuts. Eating such foods therefore engages the motivational circuits in the brain in a very powerful way and can lead to significant cravings and overconsumption.

Pornography

- The same neural circuits that motivate us to eat high-calorie foods also motivate us to be fruitful and multiply. These circuits reward us handsomely whenever we engage in sex, and they motivate us to do so. Again, this is one of the things our reward circuit was designed for. After all, if we weren't motivated to have sex, we might not have any children.

- Our brains are adapted to an environment in which sexually provocative stimuli are rare. After all, before magazines, televisions, and computers, it was actually pretty rare to see someone without any clothes on unless you were married.

- Of course, everything has changed in modern Western culture. In today's culture, we're inundated with images of naked or nearly naked people. In fact, two out of every three shows on television today include significant sexual content. And that proportion only increases during prime time. Ten percent of today's shows either depict or strongly imply sexual intercourse.

- And television is nothing compared to pornography. Getting reliable statistics on pornography is difficult, but consider these facts: In 2005, pornography accounted for approximately 70 percent of the total pay-per-view Internet content market. An analysis of 400 million Web searches between July 2009 and July 2010 found that 13 percent were looking for erotic content. Another study examined the most-common query terms on a single day in 2006 and found that 21 of the 25 most-common terms in image searches were sexual.

- As these numbers suggest, the pornography industry is an incredibly big business. In fact, in 2007, worldwide pornography revenues were estimated to be about 20 billion dollars. That's larger than the annual revenue of Netflix, Yahoo, and the National Football League combined.

- Clearly, porn is another example of a modern-day supernormal stimulus. In fact, it may be even more stimulating and rewarding than junk food. Whereas in simpler times it would be relatively rare to see sexually provocative stimuli, now it's as simple as a click of your mouse.

Video Games
- Video games have come a long way since Atari introduced the very simple tennis game Pong in the 1970s. Today's games involve sophisticated graphics, elaborate and detailed fantasy worlds, and extensive quests and adventures. And the video game industry is a very big business. For example, the game Grand Theft Auto 5 earned more than one billion dollars—in the first three days it was for sale. By comparison, that's more than five times faster than any movie in history.

- Scientific studies of video gaming are still in their infancy, but there is a growing consensus that modern video games can lead to compulsive use in some individuals. For example, Dr. Douglas Gentile at Iowa State University surveyed nearly 1,200 American kids between the ages of 8 and 18 about their use of video games.

- He found that about 8 percent of American kids met at least 6 of the criteria for pathological video game use and could be tentatively classified as pathological gamers. These kids played video games an average of about 25 hours per week and experienced significantly more problems as a result of their gaming than the other kids did.

- In extreme cases, the negative consequences can be tragic. But much like gambling, most people who play video games can do so with enough self-control that they don't lose their job and their family—or, worse, their life. At the very least, video games can be extremely engrossing. But why?

- Video game designer Michael Astolfi wrote a thesis at New York University that identified many features of modern video games that are supernormal. The basic argument is that before the development of commercial agriculture, refrigeration, and shipping, people had to hunt and forage for food for themselves and their family, so at a fairly primitive level, we may be designed to hunt and to find hunting rewarding. And modern video games take hunting to a whole new level.

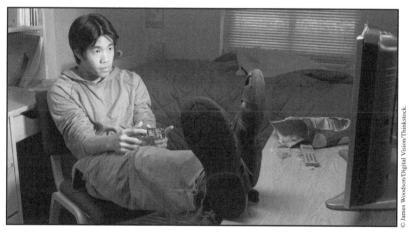

Scientific studies of video gaming are still in their infancy, but there is a growing consensus that modern video games can lead to compulsive use in some individuals.

- For example, hitting a target with a projectile is one of the core skills involved in hunting, and people also find it inherently rewarding. So, perhaps it's not a coincidence that some of the most popular and engrossing video games are first-person shooter games, which involve trying to hit targets with projectiles.

- Furthermore, in most first-person shooter games, there are a large number of targets to shoot at almost all the time. A skilled player is therefore constantly being rewarded with a hit on the order of every few seconds. Contrasting that to real hunting, particularly if you're using a primitive projectile weapon, hitting a target might happen only once every few days.

- Once again, we see how the modern stimulus is supernormal. It takes a naturally rewarding behavior and jacks it up to be significantly more stimulating than the original behavior was. And the huge video game industry is evidence of just how rewarding and engrossing that supernormal stimulus can be.

Neural Effects of Supernormal Stimuli

- Are the neural effects of supernormal stimuli similar to the effects of drugs of abuse? Scientific studies of this question are still in their infancy. In particular, neuroscientific studies of porn addiction are very few and far between. There are, however, some new studies on the neuroscience of compulsive eating and compulsive video gaming that shed some light on how these stimuli affect the brain.

- Recall that dopamine is the molecule that's associated with wanting or craving, and it underlies our motivation to do virtually everything we do—and that includes eating. Kent Berridge at the University of Michigan compared the behavior of normal mice to that of mice that had been genetically engineered to have abnormally high dopamine levels. He found that increased dopamine levels led to increased food craving.

- Dopamine also has been found to play an important role in video game playing. Matthias Koepp and his colleagues at the Hammersmith Hospital in London used positron emission tomography to measure dopamine levels in the reward circuit while participants played video games. They found that playing a simple tank navigation game led to significant increases in dopamine in the reward circuit. Furthermore, people who had the most success when playing the game also released the most dopamine.

- A second important point about the neuroscience of addiction is that the pleasure response can become numbed by repeated activation. Over time, addicts often feel less pleasure from the same dosage of their drug. Addicts often turn to larger doses of their drug in an effort to overcome their numbed experience. But doing so only further numbs the pleasure centers.

- It turns out that the same process can happen for supernormal stimuli. Ashley Gearhardt at the University of Michigan used fMRI to measure the neural response to food and food cues in two groups of young women: potential food addicts and controls. Her results are consistent with the idea that compulsive eaters are hypersensitive to food-related cues, but actually derive less-than-normal pleasure from real food consumption. This is the same kind of pattern we've seen in drug addicts: They crave drugs more despite deriving less and less pleasure from them.

- Simone Kühn and Jürgen Gallinat reported a similar finding in a neuroimaging study of pornography. Sixty-four German men were asked how much pornography they watched on average each week, and their neural activity was also measured while they viewed pornographic images. The men who watched the most pornography each week exhibited the least neural activity in the reward circuit, which is consistent with the idea that they had developed a tolerance to sexually provocative images and a numbed reward response.

- Finally, what about neural rewiring with regard to drugs of abuse? Recall that drug addiction is associated with stronger neural associations between drug-related cues and drug-taking behavior. For the drug addict, the cues might be things like a needle or a crack pipe, and these stimuli become so strongly associated with drug taking that the mere sight of them immediately triggers thoughts of getting high.

- Environmental cues can also become strongly associated with consuming junk food, viewing porn, or playing video games. For example, many people have developed very strong associations between watching television and eating high-calorie food. Stress is also a very common trigger to eat. In the case of pornography, cues could include a specific computer or sexually provocative stimuli on television or in magazines. For video games, triggers might include the sight of the game console or bumping into another regular gamer.

- Studies have confirmed these kinds of effects at a neural level. For example, Chih-Hung Ko and colleagues at the Kaohsiung Medical University in Taiwan found that game-related cues, specifically screen shots from video games, produced significantly greater reward circuit activity in the gamers than in the controls. Furthermore, participants who exhibited the most neural activity were also the ones who reported the most craving to play after viewing the pictures.

Approaches to Overcoming Behavioral Addictions
- There aren't many scientific studies on how to treat behavioral addictions yet, but a few general principles can be drawn from studies of addiction that might be helpful. First, someone with a behavioral addiction has to recognize that he or she has a problem and be committed to trying to overcome it. The motivation has to come from within; it can't come from someone else.

- Second, it's important to understand the cognitive and emotional motivations that lead to the behavior. What thoughts and feelings trigger a desire to eat junk food, view porn, play video games, or engage in any other harmful behavior? Are there particular environmental stimuli that tend to trigger the problem behavior? Once the triggers have been identified, the addict can develop a strategy for avoiding them or coping with them when they do arise.

- Third, developing a network of people to provide support and accountability can be very beneficial. Breaking an addiction requires hard work, but having a social support network can make it somewhat easier.

Suggested Reading

Barrett, *Supernormal Stimuli.*

Grant, Potenza, Weinstein, and Gorelick, "Introduction to Behavioral Addictions."

Moss, *Salt Sugar Fat.*

Wilson, "Your Brain on Porn."

Zimbardo and Duncan, *The Demise of Guys.*

Questions to Consider

1. What is a supernormal stimulus?

2. In what sense are junk food, porn, and video games supernormal?

3. Do you think that it's helpful or harmful to classify the compulsive consumption of junk food, porn, and video games as addictions?

Bibliography

Akil, Huda, Stanley J. Watson, Elizabeth Young, Michael E. Lewis, Henry Khachaturian, and J. Michael Walker. "Endogenous Opioids: Biology and Function." *Annual Review of Neuroscience* 7 (1984): 223–55.

American Psychiatric Association. *Diagnostic and Statistical Manual of Mental Disorders.* 5th ed. Arlington, VA: American Psychiatric Publishing, 2013.

Astolfi, Michael T. "The Evolutionary Psychology of Video Games: The Digital Game as Supernormal Stimulus." New York: New York University, 2012.

Avena, Nicole M., Pedro Rada, and Bartley G. Hoebel. "Evidence for Sugar Addiction: Behavioral and Neurochemical Effects of Intermittent, Excessive Sugar Intake." *Neuroscience and Biobehavioral Reviews* 32, no. 1 (2008): 20–39.

Barrett, Deirdre. *Supernormal Stimuli: How Primal Urges Overran Their Evolutionary Purpose.* New York: W. W. Norton & Company, 2010.

Berridge, Kent C. "Food Reward: Brain Substrates of Wanting and Liking." *Neuroscience and Biobehavioral Reviews* 20, no. 1 (Spring 1996): 1–25.

———. "'Liking' and 'Wanting' Food Rewards: Brain Substrates and Roles in Eating Disorders." *Physiology & Behavior* 97, no. 5 (Jul 2009): 537–550.

———. "From Prediction Error to Incentive Salience: Mesolimbic Computation of Reward Motivation." *European Journal of Neuroscience* 35, no. 7 (Apr 2012): 1124–1143.

Berridge, Kent C., Chao-Yi Ho, Jocelyn M. Richard, and Alexandra G. DiFeliceantonio. "The Tempted Brain Eats: Pleasure and Desire Circuits in Obesity and Eating Disorders." *Brain Research* 1350 (Sep 2010): 43–64.

Berridge, Kent C., Terry E. Robinson, and J. Wayne Aldridge. "Dissecting Components of Reward: 'Liking,' 'Wanting,' and Learning." *Current Opinion in Pharmacology* 9, no. 1 (Feb 2009): 65–73.

Blum, Kenneth. *Alcohol and the Addictive Brain*. New York: The Free Press, 1991.

Blum, Kenneth, John G. Cull, Eric R. Braverman, and David E. Comings. "Reward Deficiency Syndrome." *American Scientist* 84, no. 2 (Mar–Apr 1996): 132–145.

Blum, Kenneth, Peter J. Sheridan, Robert C. Wood, Eric R. Braverman, Thomas J. H. Chen, John G. Cull, and David E. Comings. "The D-2 Dopamine Receptor Gene as a Determinant of Reward Deficiency Syndrome." *Journal of the Royal Society of Medicine* 89, no. 7 (Jul 1996): 396–400.

Boecker, Henning, Till Sprenger, Mary E. Spilker, Gjermund Henriksen, Marcus Koppenhoefer, Klaus J. Wagner, Michael Valet, Achim Berthele, and Thomas R. Tolle. "The Runner's High: Opioidergic Mechanisms in the Human Brain." *Cerebral Cortex* 18, no. 11 (Nov 2008): 2523–2531.

Bryan, Cyril P. *The Papyrus Ebers*. London: The Garden City Press Ltd., 1930.

Center for Substance Abuse Treatment. "How Stimulants Affect the Brain and Behavior." In *Treatment for Stimulant Use Disorders*, edited by Substance Abuse and Mental Health Services Administration (SAMHSA), 1999. http://www.ncbi.nlm.nih.gov/books/NBK64328/.

Chavkin, Charles, Iain F. James, and Avram Goldstein. "Dynorphin Is a Specific Endogenous Ligand of the Kappa-Opioid Receptor." *Science* 215, no. 4531 (1982): 413–415.

Christie, Macdonald J. "Cellular Neuroadaptations to Chronic Opioids: Tolerance, Withdrawal and Addiction." *British Journal of Pharmacology* 154, no. 2 (May 2008): 384–396.

Comings, D. E., and K. Blum. "Reward Deficiency Syndrome: Genetic Aspects of Behavioral Disorders." In *Cognition, Emotion and Autonomic Responses: The Integrative Role of the Prefrontal Cortex and Limbic Structures*. Progress in Brain Research, 325–341, 2000.

Compton, William M., Bridget F. Grant, James D. Colliver, Meyer D. Glantz, and Frederick S. Stinson. "Prevalence of Marijuana Use Disorders in the United States: 1991–1992 and 2001–2002." *Journal of the American Medical Association* 291, no. 17 (May 5, 2004): 2114–2121.

Conyers, Beverly. *Addict in the Family: Stories of Loss, Hope, and Recovery*. Center City, MN: Hazelden, 2003.

Crabbe, John C. "Genetic Contributions to Addiction." *Annual Review of Psychology* 53 (2002): 435–462.

————. "Neurogenetic Studies of Alcohol Addiction." *Philosophical Transactions of the Royal Society B-Biological Sciences* 363, no. 1507 (Oct 2008): 3201–3211.

Crockford, David N., Bradley Goodyear, Jodi Edwards, Jeremy Quickfall, and Nady el-Guebaly. "Cue-Induced Brain Activity in Pathological Gamblers." *Biological Psychiatry* 58, no. 10 (Nov 2005): 787–795.

Dennis, Michael, Susan H. Godley, Guy Diamond, Frank M. Tims, Thomas Babor, Jean Donaldson, Howard Liddle, et al. "The Cannabis Youth Treatment (CYT) Study: Main Findings from Two Randomized Trials." *Journal of Substance Abuse Treatment* 27, no. 3 (Oct 2004): 197–213.

Deroche-Gamonet, Veronique, David Belin, and Pier Vincenzo Piazza. "Evidence for Addiction-Like Behavior in the Rat." *Science* 305, no. 5686 (Aug 2004): 1014–1017.

Devane, William A., Francis A. Dysarz, M. Ross Johnson, Lawrence S. Melvin, and Allyn C. Howlett. "Determination and Characterization of a Cannabinoid Receptor in Rat-Brain." *Molecular Pharmacology* 34, no. 5 (Nov 1988): 605–613.

Devane, William A., Lumir Hanus, Aviva Breuer, Roger G. Pertwee, Lesley A. Stevenson, Graeme Griffin, Dan Gibson, et al. "Isolation and Structure of a Brain Constituent That Binds to the Cannabinoid Receptor." *Science* 258, no. 5090 (Dec 18, 1992): 1946–1949.

Di Chiara, Gaetano, and Assunta Imperato. "Drugs Abused by Humans Preferentially Increase Synaptic Dopamine Concentrations in the Mesolimbic System of Freely Moving Rats." *Proceedings of the National Academy of Sciences of the United States of America* 85, no. 14 (Jul 1988): 5274–5278.

Drgon, Tomas, Ping-Wu Zhang, Catherine Johnson, Donna Walther, Judith Hess, Michelle Nino, and George R. Uhl. "Genome Wide Association for Addiction: Replicated Results and Comparisons of Two Analytic Approaches." *PLoS One* 5, no. 1 (Jan 21, 2010): e8832. doi: 10.1371/journal.pone.0008832.

Earleywine, Mitch. *Understanding Marijuana: A New Look at the Scientific Evidence*. New York: Oxford University Press, 2002.

Eisen, Seth A., Nong Lin, Michael J. Lyons, Jeffrey F. Scherrer, Kristin Griffith, William R. True, Jack Goldberg, and Ming T. Tsuang. "Familial Influences on Gambling Behavior: An Analysis of 3359 Twin Pairs." *Addiction* 93, no. 9 (Sep 1998): 1375–1384.

el-Guebaly, Nady, Tanya Mudry, Joseph Zohar, Hermano Tavares, and Marc N. Potenza. "Compulsive Features in Behavioural Addictions: The Case of Pathological Gambling." *Addiction* 107, no. 10 (Oct 2012): 1726–1734.

Erickson, Carlton K. *The Science of Addiction: From Neurobiology to Treatment*. New York: W. W. Norton & Company, 2007.

Escohotado, Antonio. *A Brief History of Drugs: From the Stone Age to the Stoned Age*. Rochester, VT: Park Street Press, 1999.

Everitt, Barry J., and Trevor W. Robbins. "Neural Systems of Reinforcement for Drug Addiction: From Actions to Habits to Compulsion." *Nature Neuroscience* 8, no. 11 (Nov 2005): 1481–1489.

Fernandez, Humberto, and Therissa A. Libby. *Heroin: Its History, Pharmacology & Treatment*. 2nd ed. Center City, MN: Hazelden, 2011.

Fredholm, Bertil B., Karl Battig, Janet Holmen, Astrid Nehlig, and Edwin E. Zvartau. "Actions of Caffeine in the Brain with Special Reference to Factors That Contribute to Its Widespread Use." *Pharmacological Reviews* 51, no. 1 (Mar 1999): 83–133.

Gately, Iain. *Drink: A Cultural History of Alcohol*. New York: Gotham Books, 2008.

Gearhardt, Ashley N., William R. Corbin, and Kelly D. Brownell. "Preliminary Validation of the Yale Food Addiction Scale." *Appetite* 52, no. 2 (Apr 2009): 430–436.

———. "Food Addiction: An Examination of the Diagnostic Criteria for Dependence." *Journal of Addiction Medicine* 3, no. 1 (Mar 2009): 1–7.

Gearhardt, Ashley N., Sonja Yokum, Patrick T. Orr, Eric Stice, William R. Corbin, and Kelly D. Brownell. "Neural Correlates of Food Addiction." *Archives of General Psychiatry* 68, no. 8 (Aug 2011): 808–816.

Genetic Science Learning Center. The University of Utah. "The New Science of Addiction: Genetics and the Brain." http://learn.genetics.utah.edu/content/addiction/.

Gentile, Douglas. "Pathological Video-Game Use among Youth Ages 8 to 18: A National Study." *Psychological Science* 20, no. 5 (May 2009): 594–602.

Goudriaan, Anna E., and L. Clark. "Neuroimaging in Problem Gambling." In *Biological Research on Addiction: Comprehensive Addictive Behaviors and Disorders*, Vol 2, 689–697, 2013.

Goudriaan, Anna E., Michiel B. de Ruiter, Wim van den Brink, Jaap Oosterlaan, and Dick J. Veltman. "Brain Activation Patterns Associated with Cue Reactivity and Craving in Abstinent Problem Gamblers, Heavy Smokers and Healthy Controls: An fMRI Study." *Addiction Biology* 15, no. 4 (Oct 2010): 491–503.

Goudriaan, Anna E., Jaap Oosterlaan, Edwin de Beurs, and Wim van den Brink. "Pathological Gambling: A Comprehensive Review of Biobehavioral Findings." *Neuroscience and Biobehavioral Reviews* 28, no. 2 (Apr 2004): 123–141.

———. "Decision Making in Pathological Gambling: A Comparison between Pathological Gamblers, Alcohol Dependents, Persons with Tourette Syndrome, and Normal Controls." *Cognitive Brain Research* 23, no. 1 (Apr 2005): 137–151.

———. "Neurocognitive Functions in Pathological Gambling: A Comparison with Alcohol Dependence, Tourette Syndrome and Normal Controls." *Addiction* 101, no. 4 (Apr 2006): 534–547.

Goudriaan, Anna E., Ruth J. van Holst, Dick J. Veltman, and Wim van den Brink. "Betting on the Brain: Neuroimaging Research in Pathological Gambling, Similarities and Differences with Substance Use Disorders." *Substance Abuse* 34, no. 3 (Jul 2013): 326–327.

Grant, Jon E., Judson A. Brewer, and Marc N. Potenza. "The Neurobiology of Substance and Behavioral Addictions." *CNS Spectrums* 11, no. 12 (Dec 2006): 924–930.

Grant, Jon E., and Marc N. Potenza, eds. *Pathological Gambling: A Clinical Guide to Treatment*. Arlington, VA: American Psychiatric Publishing, 2004.

Grant, Jon E., Marc N. Potenza, Aviv Weinstein, and David A. Gorelick. "Introduction to Behavioral Addictions." *American Journal of Drug and Alcohol Abuse* 36, no. 5 (Sep 2010): 233–241.

Griffiths, Mark. "Tolerance in Gambling: An Objective-Measure Using the Psychophysiological Analysis of Male Fruit Machine Gamblers." *Addictive Behaviors* 18, no. 3 (May–Jun 1993): 365–372.

Guzman, Manuel. "Cannabinoids: Potential Anticancer Agents." *Nature Reviews Cancer* 3, no. 10 (Oct 2003): 745–755.

Heath, Robert G. "Electrical Self-Stimulation of the Brain in Man." *American Journal of Psychiatry* 120, no. 6 (1963): 571–577.

Hilton, Donald L. "Pornography Addiction: A Supranormal Stimulus Considered in the Context of Neuroplasticity." *Socioaffective Neuroscience & Psychology* 3 (2013): 20767–20774.

Hyman, Steven E., and Robert C. Malenka. "Addiction and the Brain: The Neurobiology of Compulsion and Its Persistence." *Nature Reviews Neuroscience* 2, no. 10 (Oct 2001): 695–703.

Iversen, Leslie. "Cannabis and the Brain." *Brain* 126 (Jun 2003): 1252–1270.

Iverson, Leslie I. *The Science of Marijuana.* 2nd ed. New York: Oxford University Press, 2008.

Jentsch, J. David, and Jane R. Taylor. "Impulsivity Resulting from Frontostriatal Dysfunction in Drug Abuse: Implications for the Control of Behavior by Reward-Related Stimuli." *Psychopharmacology* 146, no. 4 (Oct 1999): 373–390.

Johnson, Bankole A., ed. *Addiction Medicine: Science and Practice.* Vol. 1. New York: Springer, 2011.

Johnson, Paul M., and Paul J. Kenny. "Dopamine D2 Receptors in Addiction-Like Reward Dysfunction and Compulsive Eating in Obese Rats." *Nature Neuroscience* 13, no. 5 (May 2010): 635–U156.

Bibliography

Kalivas, Peter W., and Nora D. Volkow. "The Neural Basis of Addiction: A Pathology of Motivation and Choice." *American Journal of Psychiatry* 162, no. 8 (Aug 2005): 1403–1413.

Ketcham, Katherine, William F. Asbury, Mel Schulstad, and Arthur P. Ciaramicoli. *Beyond the Influence: Understanding and Defeating Alcoholism.* New York: Bantam Books, 2000.

Koob, George F. "Drugs of Abuse: Anatomy, Pharmacology and Function of Reward Pathways." *Trends in Pharmacological Sciences* 13, no. 5 (May 1992): 177–184.

Koob, George F., and Floyd E. Bloom. "Cellular and Molecular Mechanisms of Drug-Dependence." *Science* 242, no. 4879 (Nov 4, 1988): 715–723.

Kranzier, Henry R., Domenic A. Ciraulo, and Leah R. Zindel, eds. *Clinical Manual of Addiction Psychopharmacology.* 2nd ed. Arlington, VA: American Psychiatric Publishing, 2013.

Kringelbach, Morten L., and Kent C. Berridge. "Towards a Functional Neuroanatomy of Pleasure and Happiness." *Trends in Cognitive Sciences* 13, no. 11 (Nov 2009): 479–487.

———. "The Joyful Mind." *Scientific American* 307, no. 2 (Aug 2012): 40–45.

Leeman, Robert F., and Marc N. Potenza. "A Targeted Review of the Neurobiology and Genetics of Behavioural Addictions: An Emerging Area of Research." *Canadian Journal of Psychiatry-Revue Canadienne De Psychiatrie* 58, no. 5 (May 2013): 260–273.

Li, Ming D., and Margit Burmeister. "New Insights into the Genetics of Addiction." *Nature Reviews Genetics* 10, no. 4 (Apr 2009): 225–231.

Liu, Timothy, and Marc N. Potenza. "Problematic Internet Use: Clinical Implications." *CNS Spectrums* 12, no. 6 (Jun 2007): 453–466.

Lobo, Daniela S. S., and James L. Kennedy. "Genetic Aspects of Pathological Gambling: A Complex Disorder with Shared Genetic Vulnerabilities." *Addiction* 104, no. 9 (Sep 2009): 1454–1465.

Luttinger, Nina, and Gregory Dicum. *The Coffee Book: Anatomy of an Industry from Crop to the Last Drop*. New York: The New Press, 2006.

Lynskey, Michael T., Andrew C. Heath, Kathleen K. Bucholz, Wendy S. Slutske, Pamela A. F. Madden, Elliot C. Nelson, Dixie J. Statham, and Nicholas G. Martin. "Escalation of Drug Use in Early-Onset Cannabis Users Vs. Co-Twin Controls." *Journal of the American Medical Association* 289, no. 4 (Jan 22, 2003): 427–433.

Markel, Howard. *An Anatomy of Addiction: Sigmund Freud, William Halsted, and the Miracle Drug Cocaine*. New York: Pantheon Books, 2011.

Marsicano, Giovanni, Carsten T. Wotjak, Shahnaz C. Azad, Tiziana Bisogno, Gerhard Rammes, Maria Grazia Cascio, Heike Hermann, et al. "The Endogenous Cannabinoid System Controls Extinction of Aversive Memories." *Nature* 418, no. 6897 (Aug 1, 2002): 530–534.

Martin, Steven. *Opium Fiend: A 21st Century Slave to a 19th Century Addiction*. New York: Villard Books, 2012.

Matthes, Hans W. D., Rafael Maldonado, Frederic Simonin, Olga Valverde, Susan Slowe, Ian Kitchen, Katia Befort, et al. "Loss of Morphine-Induced Analgesia, Reward Effect and Withdrawal Symptoms in Mice Lacking the Mu-Opioid-Receptor Gene." *Nature* 383, no. 6603 (Oct 31, 1996): 819–823.

Mayo Clinic. "Nicotine Dependence." http://www.mayoclinic.com/health/nicotine-dependence/DS00307/DSECTION=treatments-and-drugs.

McCabe, Sean Esteban, Christian J. Teter, and Carol J. Boyd. "Medical Use, Illicit Use, and Diversion of Abusable Prescription Drugs." *Journal of American College Health* 54, no. 5 (Mar–Apr 2006): 269–278.

Bibliography

McClearn, Gerald E., and David A. Rodgers. "Genetic Factors in Alcohol Preference of Laboratory Mice." *Journal of Comparative and Physiological Psychology* 54, no. 2 (1961): 116–119.

McGovern, Patrick E., Juzhong Zhang, Jigen Tang, Zhiqing Zhang, Gretchen R. Hall, Robert A. Moreau, Alberto Nunez, et al. "Fermented Beverages of Pre- and Proto-Historic China." *Proceedings of the National Academy of Sciences of the United States of America* 101, no. 51 (Dec 21, 2004): 17593–17598.

Meyer, Jerrold S., and Linda F. Quenzer. *Psychopharmacology: Drugs, the Brain, and Behavior*. 2nd ed. Sunderland, MA: Sinauer Associates Inc., 2013.

Moore, Elaine A. *The Amphetamine Debate: The Use of Adderall, Ritalin and Related Drugs for Behavior Modification, Neuroenhancement and Anti-Aging Purposes*. Jefferson, NC: McFarland & Company Inc., 2010.

Moss, Michael. *Salt Sugar Fat: How the Food Giants Hooked Us*. New York: Random House, 2013.

Nash, J. Madeleine. "Addicted: Why Do People Get Hooked?" *Time Magazine*. May 5, 1997. http://content.time.com/time/magazine/article/0,9171,986282,00.html.

National Cancer Institute. "Smokefree.Gov." http://smokefree.gov.

———. "Tobacco Statistics." http://www.cancer.gov/cancertopics/tobacco/statisticsresources.

National Institute on Drug Abuse. "Trends and Statistics." http://www.drugabuse.gov/related-topics/trends-statistics.

———. "Drugs and the Brain." http://www.drugabuse.gov/publications/drugs-brains-behavior-science-addiction/drugs-brain.

———. *Drugs, Brains, and Behavior: The Science of Addiction*. 2010. http://www.drugabuse.gov/sites/default/files/sciofaddiction.pdf.

Nehlig, Astrid. "Are We Dependent upon Coffee and Caffeine? A Review on Human and Animal Data." *Neuroscience and Biobehavioral Reviews* 23, no. 4 (Mar 1999): 563–576.

Nehlig, Astrid, Jean-Luc Daval, and Gerard Debry. "Caffeine and the Central Nervous System: Mechanisms of Action, Biochemical, Metabolic and Psychostimulant Effects." *Brain Research Reviews* 17, no. 2 (May–Aug 1992): 139–169.

Nestler, Eric J., Steven E. Hyman, and Robert C. Malenka. *Molecular Neuropharmacology: A Foundation for Clinical Neuroscience.* New York: McGraw-Hill, 2009.

Nestler, Eric J., and Robert C. Malenka. "The Addicted Brain." *Scientific American* 290, no. 3 (Mar 2004): 78–85.

Nolte, John. *The Human Brain: An Introduction to Its Functional Anatomy.* 6th ed. Philadelphia, PA: Mosby Elsevier, 2009.

Olds, James, and Peter Milner. "Positive Reinforcement Produced by Electrical Stimulation of Septal Area and Other Regions of Rat Brain." *Journal of Comparative and Physiological Psychology* 47, no. 6 (1954): 419–427.

Pecina, Susana, and Kent C. Berridge. "Opioid Site in Nucleus Accumbens Shell Mediates Eating and Hedonic 'Liking' for Food: Map Based on Microinjection FOS Plumes." *Brain Research* 863, nos. 1–2 (Apr 2000): 71–86.

———. "Hedonic Hot Spot in Nucleus Accumbens Shell: Where Do Mu-Opioids Cause Increased Hedonic Impact of Sweetness?" *Journal of Neuroscience* 25, no. 50 (Dec 2005): 11777–11786.

Pecina, Susana, Kyle S. Smith, and Kent C. Berridge. "Hedonic Hot Spots in the Brain." *Neuroscientist* 12, no. 6 (Dec 2006): 500–511.

Petrovic, Predrag, Eija Kalso, Karl Magnus Petersson, and Martin Ingvar. "Placebo and Opioid Analgesia: Imaging a Shared Neuronal Network." *Science* 295, no. 5560 (Mar 1, 2002): 1737–1740.

Potenza, Marc N. "Should Addictive Disorders Include Non-Substance-Related Conditions?" *Addiction* 101 (Sep 2006): 142–151.

———. "The Neurobiology of Pathological Gambling and Drug Addiction: An Overview and New Findings." *Philosophical Transactions of the Royal Society B-Biological Sciences* 363, no. 1507 (Oct 2008): 3181–3189.

———. "Neurobiology of Gambling Behaviors." *Current Opinion in Neurobiology* 23, no. 4 (Aug 2013): 660–667.

Potenza, Marc N., Hoi-Chung Leung, Hilary P. Blumberg, Bradley S. Peterson, Robert K. Fulbright, Cheryl M. Lacadie, Pawel Skudlarski, and John C. Gore. "An fMRI Stroop Task Study of Ventromedial Prefrontal Cortical Function in Pathological Gamblers." *American Journal of Psychiatry* 160, no. 11 (Nov 2003): 1990–1994.

Potenza, Marc N., Marvin A. Steinberg, Pawel Skudlarski, Robert K. Fulbright, Cheryl M. Lacadie, Mary K. Wilber, Bruce J. Rounsaville, John C. Gore, and Bruce E. Wexler. "Gambling Urges in Pathological Gambling: A Functional Magnetic Resonance Imaging Study." *Archives of General Psychiatry* 60, no. 8 (Aug 2003): 828–836.

Powell, Russell A., P. Lynne Honey, and Diane G. Symbaluk. *Introduction to Learning and Behavior*. Belmont, CA: Wadsworth, 2013.

Proctor, Robert N. *Golden Holocaust: Origins of the Cigarette Catastrophe and the Case for Abolition*. Berkeley: University of California Press, 2011.

Rada, Pedro, Nicole M. Avena, and Bartley G. Hoebel. "Daily Bingeing on Sugar Repeatedly Releases Dopamine in the Accumbens Shell." *Neuroscience* 134, no. 3 (2005): 737–744.

Redish, A. David. "Addiction as a Computational Process Gone Awry." *Science* 306, no. 5703 (Dec 2004): 1944–1947.

Redish, A. David. *The Mind within the Brain: How We Make Decisions and How Those Decisions Go Wrong*. New York: Oxford University Press, 2013.

Redish, A. David, Steve Jensen, and Adam Johnson. "A Unified Framework for Addiction: Vulnerabilities in the Decision Process." *Behavioral and Brain Sciences* 31, no. 4 (Aug 2008): 415–437.

Redish, A. David, Steve Jensen, Adam Johnson, and Zeb Kurth-Nelson. "Reconciling Reinforcement Learning Models with Behavioral Extinction and Renewal: Implications for Addiction, Relapse, and Problem Gambling." *Psychological Review* 114, no. 3 (Jul 2007): 784–805.

Rescorla, Robert A., and Allan R. Wagner. "A Theory of Pavlovian Conditioning: Variations in the Effectiveness of Reinforcement and Nonreinforcement." In *Classical Conditioning Ii: Current Theory and Research*, edited by A. H. Black and W. F. Prokasy. New York: Appleton-Century-Crofts, 1972.

Research Triangle Institute. "National Survey on Drug Use and Health." https://nsduhweb.rti.org/.

Reuter, Jan, Thomas Raedler, Michael Rose, Iver Hand, Jan Glascher, and Christian Buchel. "Pathological Gambling Is Linked to Reduced Activation of the Mesolimbic Reward System." *Nature Neuroscience* 8, no. 2 (Feb 2005): 147–148.

Ridley, Matt. *The Agile Gene: How Nature Turns on Nurture*. New York: Perennial, 2004.

Robinson, Terry E., and Kent C. Berridge. "The Neural Basis of Drug Craving: An Incentive-Sensitization Theory of Addiction." *Brain Research Reviews* 18, no. 3 (Sep–Dec 1993): 247–291.

———. "Addiction." *Annual Review of Psychology* 54 (2003): 25–53.

Santangelo, Gabriella, Paolo Barone, Luigi Trojano, and Carmine Vitale. "Pathological Gambling in Parkinson's Disease: A Comprehensive Review." *Parkinsonism & Related Disorders* 19, no. 7 (Jul 2013): 645–653.

Schüll, Natasha Dow. *Addiction by Design: Machine Gambling in Las Vegas*. Princeton, NJ: Princeton University Press, 2012.

Schultz, Wolfram, Peter Dayan, and P. Read Montague. "A Neural Substrate of Prediction and Reward." *Science* 275, no. 5306 (1997): 1593–1599.

Sheff, David. *Beautiful Boy: A Father's Journey through His Son's Addiction*. New York: Houghton Mifflin Harcourt, 2008.

Sheff, David. *Clean: Overcoming Addiction and Ending America's Greatest Tragedy*. New York: Houghton Mifflin Harcourt Publishing, 2013.

Snyder, Solomon H. *Drugs and the Brain*. Scientific American Library Series. New York: W. H. Freeman & Co., 1996.

Steeves, T. D. L., J. Miyasaki, M. Zurowski, A. E. Lang, G. Pellecchia, T. Van Eimeren, P. Rusjan, S. Houle, and A. P. Strafella. "Increased Striatal Dopamine Release in Parkinsonian Patients with Pathological Gambling: A [C-11] Raclopride Pet Study." *Brain* 132 (May 2009): 1376–1385.

Stice, Eric, Sonja Yokum, Kenneth Blum, and Cara Bohon. "Weight Gain Is Associated with Reduced Striatal Response to Palatable Food." *Journal of Neuroscience* 30, no. 39 (Sep 2010): 13105–13109.

Stoeckel, Luke E., Rosalyn E. Weller, Edwin W. Cook, III, Donald B. Twieg, Robert C. Knowlton, and James E. Cox. "Widespread Reward-System Activation in Obese Women in Response to Pictures of High-Calorie Foods." *Neuroimage* 41, no. 2 (Jun 2008): 636–647.

Sutton, Richard S., and Andrew G. Barto. *Reinforcement Learning: An Introduction*. Cambridge, MA: MIT Press, 1998.

Tesauro, Gerald. "Temporal Difference Learning and TD-Gammon." *Communications of the ACM* 38, no. 3 (1995): 58–68.

Thomasson, Holly R., Howard J. Edenberg, David W. Crabb, Xiao-Ling Mai, Ronald E. Jerome, Ting-Kai Li, Shiou-Ping Wang, et al. "Alcohol and Aldehyde Dehydrogenase Genotypes and Alcoholism in Chinese Men." *American Journal of Human Genetics* 48, no. 4 (Apr 1991): 677–681.

Uhl, George R., Tomas Drgon, Catherine Johnson, Olutuatosin O. Fatusin, Qing-Rong Liu, Carlo Contoreggi, Chuan-Yun Li, Kari Buck, and John Crabbe. "'Higher Order' Addiction Molecular Genetics: Convergent Data from Genome-Wide Association in Humans and Mice." *Biochemical Pharmacology* 75, no. 1 (Jan 2008): 98–111.

Valenstein, Eliot S. *The War of the Soups and the Sparks: The Discovery of Neurotransmitters and the Dispute over How Nerves Communicate.* New York: Columbia University Press, 2005.

van Holst, Ruth J., Wim van den Brink, Dick J. Veltman, and Anna E. Goudriaan. "Why Gamblers Fail to Win: A Review of Cognitive and Neuroimaging Findings in Pathological Gambling." *Neuroscience and Biobehavioral Reviews* 34, no. 1 (Jan 2010): 87–107.

———. "Brain Imaging Studies in Pathological Gambling." *Current Psychiatry Reports* 12, no. 5 (Oct 2010): 418–425.

Varvel, Stephen A., and Aron H. Lichtman. "Evaluation of CB1 Receptor Knockout Mice in the Morris Water Maze." *Journal of Pharmacology and Experimental Therapeutics* 301, no. 3 (Jun 2002): 915–924.

Volkow, Nora D., Joanna S. Fowler, Gene-Jack Wang, and James M. Swanson. "Dopamine in Drug Abuse and Addiction: Results from Imaging Studies and Treatment Implications." *Molecular Psychiatry* 9, no. 6 (Jun 2004): 557–569.

Volkow, Nora D., Joanna S. Fowler, Gene-Jack Wang, James M. Swanson, and Frank Telang. "Dopamine in Drug Abuse and Addiction: Results of Imaging Studies and Treatment Implications." *Archives of Neurology* 64, no. 11 (Nov 2007): 1575–1579.

Volkow, Nora D., Gene-Jack Wang, Joanna S. Fowler, and Frank Telang. "Overlapping Neuronal Circuits in Addiction and Obesity: Evidence of Systems Pathology." *Philosophical Transactions of the Royal Society B-Biological Sciences* 363, no. 1507 (Oct 2008): 3191–3200.

Volkow, Nora D., Gene-Jack Wang, Dardo Tomasi, and Ruben D. Baler. "Obesity and Addiction: Neurobiological Overlaps." *Obesity Reviews* 14, no. 1 (Jan 2013): 2–18.

Volkow, Nora D., and Roy A. Wise. "How Can Drug Addiction Help Us Understand Obesity?" *Nature Neuroscience* 8, no. 5 (May 2005): 555–560.

Wilson, Gary. "Your Brain on Porn." http://yourbrainonporn.com/.

Wise, Roy A. "Neurobiology of Addiction." *Current Opinion in Neurobiology* 6, no. 2 (Apr 1996): 243–251.

Wolff, Peter H. "Ethnic Differences in Alcohol Sensitivity." *Science* 175, no. 4020 (1972): 449–450.

Zimbardo, Philip G., and Nikita Duncan. *The Demise of Guys: Why Boys Are Struggling and What We Can Do about It.* New York: TED Conferences, 2012.

Zubieta, Jon-Kar, Joshua A. Bueller, Lisa R. Jackson, David J. Scott, Yanjun Xu, Robert A. Koeppe, Thomas E. Nichols, and Christian S. Stohler. "Placebo Effects Mediated by Endogenous Opioid Activity on Mu-Opioid Receptors." *Journal of Neuroscience* 25, no. 34 (Aug 24, 2005): 7754–7762.

Notes

Notes

Notes